Rhinoplasty

Everything You Need to Know about Fixing and Reshaping Your Nose

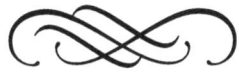

ISBN-10: 1480208892
ISBN-13: 9781480208896
Library of Congress Control Number: 2012920979
CreateSpace Independent Publishing Platform
North Charleston, South Carolina

Is Rhinoplasty for You?

With straight talk and a knack for explaining the process in easily accessible terms, Dr. Williams has written the definitive guide for those considering nose-shaping surgery.

"When I was fifteen years old, I was depressed and embarrassed by the size of my nose. I begged my mother daily to have a rhinoplasty. She said she would give me permission if I researched the surgery and prices and found a doctor. So I hand wrote letters to all the doctors in the area. Only one replied, Dr. Williams. Dr. Williams performed the surgery, and I've never been happier. It's now eleven years later and I've referred many people, who were all happy with the results."

— Sonya, Albany, New York

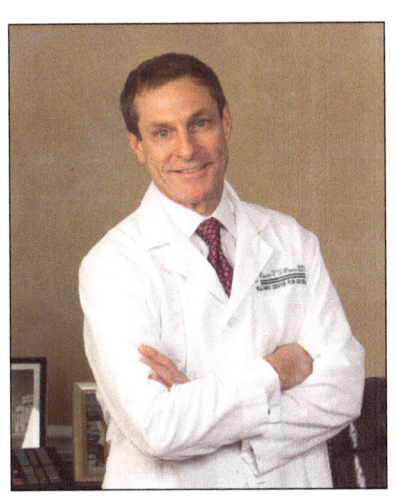

Nothing has a greater impact on how you look (and feel) than the size and shape of your nose. But is a nose job right for you? What do you need to know before deciding to have rhinoplasty surgery?

Dr. Edwin Williams, internationally recognized and respected Board Certified Facial Plastic Surgeon, answers your most frequently asked questions about rhinoplasty with the skill and intelligence of an accomplished surgeon and the compassion and understanding gained in twenty-one years of successful practice.

Dr. Williams has helped thousands of patients decide whether or not this procedure is for them. Dr. Williams has mastered this complicated yet common procedure, performing over thirty-five hundred such surgeries in his medical career.

In this guide, Dr. Williams addresses your every concern about rhinoplasty, including:

Which rhinoplasty procedure is right for me?

Is there more than one way to fix my nose?

Will it hurt?

How much will it cost?

When can I get back to work and working out?

Dr. Williams not only answers these questions, but anticipates and answers others, sharing his expertise, knowledge, and vast experience in clear and accessible language for those considering rhinoplasty.

Dedication

While there are many rhinoplasty surgeons who have mentored me and taught me the principles of rhinoplasty, it is my patients who have been my greatest teachers. They have given me countless opportunities to develop as a surgeon and a person, teaching me some of life's most valuable lessons in the process.

It is with appreciation and gratitude that I dedicate this book to all of them.

To the Victims of Domestic Violence

All proceeds from the sale of this informational guide will be donated to the FACE TO FACE program, the humanitarian and educational surgical exchange program conducted under the auspices of the Educational and Research Foundation for the American Academy of Facial Plastic and Reconstructive Surgery (AAFPRS Foundation).

FACE TO FACE is staffed by medical personnel—facial plastic and reconstructive surgeons, nurses, speech pathologists, and anesthesiologists—who donate their time and expertise, frequently for two weeks at a time. Among those they help are women in this country, where domestic violence has wreaked havoc on their lives both emotionally and physically.

http://www.aafprs.org/physician/humanitarian/ph_ffviolence.html

Thank you for your contribution.

My Journey

My journey in the field of rhinoplasty began during my surgical training, where I became more and more interested in facial trauma and the reconstructive aspects of facial plastic surgery. Over the next several years, I developed a fascination with the reconstruction and aesthetic aspects of the nose and decided to pursue a fellowship whose primary focus involved rhinoplasty and nasal reconstruction.

The complexity of nasal reconstruction surgery and its various forms continues to challenge my thinking on a daily basis. The profound impact this seemingly simple procedure can have on a patient's self-esteem and functionality continues to intrigue me, and I find this work extraordinarily fulfilling.

Special Thanks

A special thank you to the very talented people, especially the staff of the Williams Center for Plastic Surgery, who contributed to this project:

Merci Miglino, editor and writer—for her guidance and creative influence.

Susan Sullivan, RN, chief operating officer for the Williams Center—for her constant insight, guidance, and support.

Christopher Hove, MD, facial plastic surgeon and medical illustrator—for his informative and artful illustrations.

Cherie Williams, my wife, and my family, Katie, Riley, Lydia, and Evan—for their constant support and understanding, which has allowed me to achieve this next level in my rhinoplasty surgical career.

Table of Contents

Intro

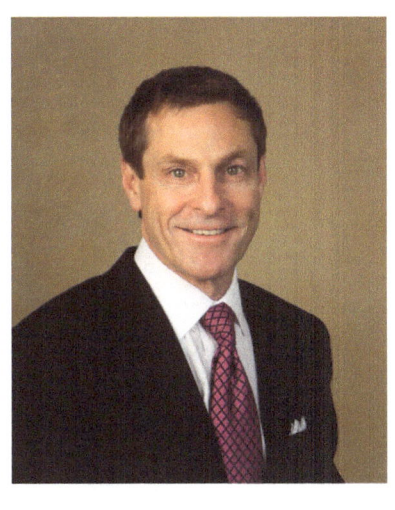

When asked my ultimate objective in performing rhinoplasty, my answer is always the same: I want to leave you with a nose you don't see.

Sounds a bit counterintuitive, right? Here we are reading a book whose entire focus is about fixing the nose, and I'm suggesting that you want a nose that you don't see.

Let me explain. There are many studies out there exploring what "visual fields" folks are looking at when they stare at, say, the *Mona Lisa* or when intently listening to another person. According to these studies, the human mind seeks to connect with the eyes of another. Applying this to the goal of rhinoplasty, we want to see the eyes and not "see" the nose. We want the nose to play second fiddle, so to speak, while the eyes take the lead.

Taking the attention away from the nose means making it so natural that when people are looking at your face or at your before-and-after photos, it's not obvious that you have had your nose fixed.

The art of facial surgery is bringing the face into balance without losing the unique characteristics that define the patient's identity. My intent in writing this book is to answer your questions about the surgery and let you in on what I, as an experienced rhinoplasty surgeon and a Board Certified Facial Plastic Surgeon, have learned over the years.

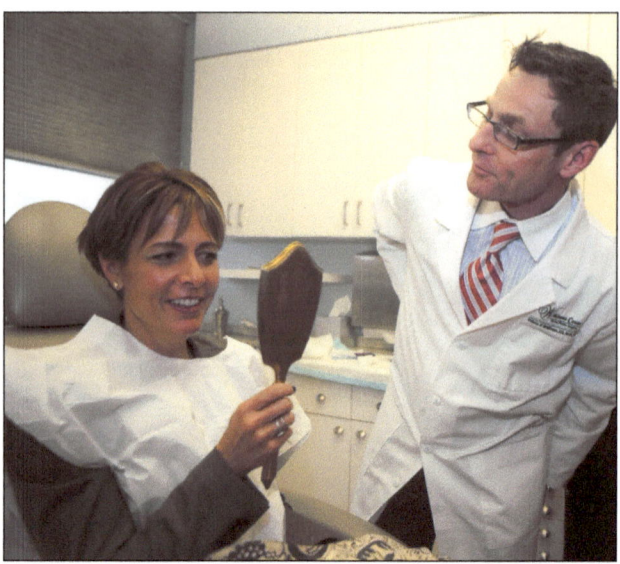

After performing this complicated yet common procedure some thirty-five hundred times, I have become especially tuned in to what patients want to know before making the decision to proceed with the surgery. The very first thing I do in my consultations, before I even share the specifics about what I see, is ask what you don't like about your nose. I listen to what is said (and not said). If you say, "I have big nostrils," that might mean one thing to you and another to me as a surgeon, so listening with the intent to really understand your concerns is essential if I am to help set and meet your expectations.

In some cases, patients may not be able to articulate their concerns. That's when I say, "Well, let me tell you what I see. I'm going to use some medical terms, but then I'm going to try to communicate them in a way that you can relate to." As I observe your nose and share what I see, I might talk about what we surgeons call "projection," which simply means the nose is too far from your face, as seen in the before-and-after photos as seen on the following page.

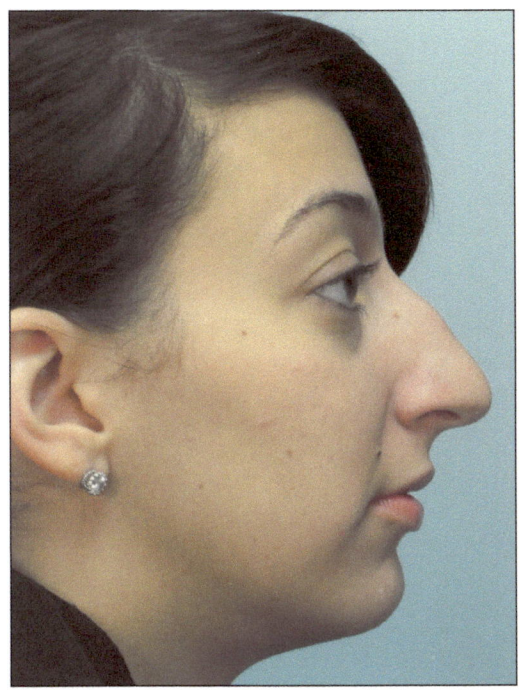 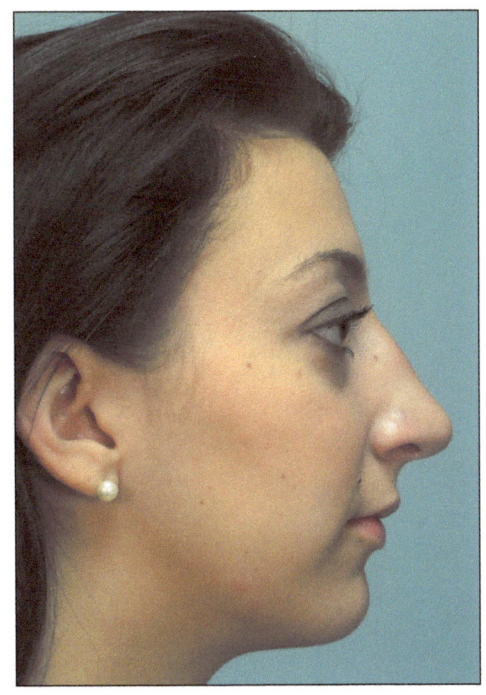

RHINOPLASTY BEFORE AND AFTER EXAMPLE

If I don't take the opportunity to *really* listen to you, I could miss an essential aspect of what changes are important to you. I understand that for many patients, it's difficult to speak up when they perceive someone's expertise as beyond theirs. However, I encourage you to speak up. Make every effort to share what you want and don't want. Give your surgeon every opportunity to meet your expectations and needs with his or her expertise and skill—the result of which is something both of you can feel great about.

My appreciation for patients' perspective and input is why I've enjoyed success as a rhinoplasty surgeon. Obviously, my hard work and resulting skill are critical, but really most of what I've learned comes from my conversations with the patients.

Chapter 1

A Nose by Any Other Shape Would Smell as Sweet

While this is a book about the aesthetic nature of the nose and what we can do to improve it, we'll start with some basic information on what your nose does and how it does it.

Simply put, the nose helps us breathe and smell. It also warms, moistens, and filters the air before it goes to the lungs.

The nose is the main entry to the respiratory system, your body's system for breathing. When you inhale through your nostrils, the air enters the nasal passages and travels into your nasal cavity. The air then passes down the back of your throat into the trachea, or windpipe, on its way to the lungs.

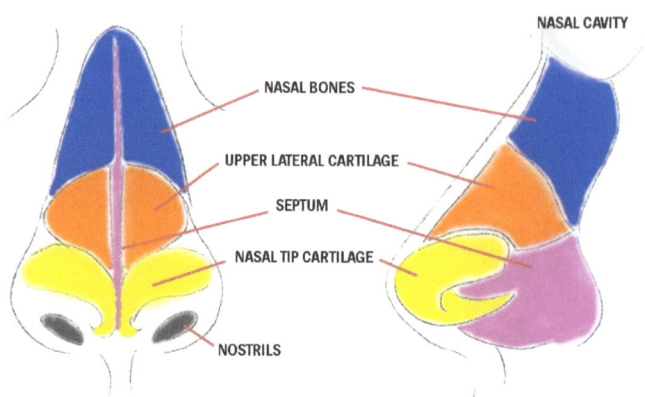

NASAL ANATOMY

The straight hollow tubes of the nostrils are shaped specifically to regulate airflow. A wall called the septum, made of very thin pieces of bone, separates the nostrils and the nasal passages.

Closer to the tip of your nose, the septum is made of cartilage, a flexible material that's firmer than skin or muscle but not as hard as bone. Behind your nose is a space called the nasal cavity, which connects with the back of the throat. The nasal cavity is separated from the inside of your mouth by the palate (roof of your mouth).

The nose also detects smells and contributes to our sense of taste. For us to smell something, molecules from that source have to make it to the nose. Everything we smell is giving off molecules, whether it's perfume, onions, or something far less pleasant. Those molecules are generally light, volatile (easily evaporated) chemicals that float through the air into your nose.

Chapter 2

Why Consider Rhinoplasty?

Every year over half a million people interested in improving the appearance of their nose seek consultation with a facial plastic surgeon. Since you are reading this book, I'm going to assume you are one of them. You may be a teen or young adult becoming more aware of your appearance. Perhaps a friend has had a rhinoplasty and you are noticing how much happier he or she is with his or her appearance. You may have suffered name calling or worse because of the size or shape of your nose.

Or maybe you are someone who finally has the time and money to get the rhinoplasty you always wanted or to explore what the surgery can do to enhance your looks or create a younger-looking and more vital appearance.

Whatever the reason for your consideration, you want to know exactly what to expect from a rhinoplasty. First, let me say that the ideal goal in rhinoplasty is to improve the nose aesthetically, making it harmonize better with other facial features so that it has a more natural, normal appearance. This way the nose will blend better with the face, rather than be the dominant or obvious feature. To give my patients the best opportunity to visualize what's possible for their unique features, and to determine if their expectations are realistic, I use a computerized imager during the initial consultation.

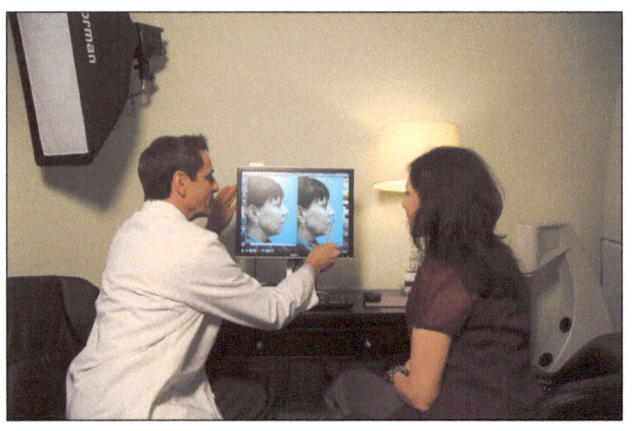

Computer-Generated Imagery (CGI) is a specialized computer program that allows me to manipulate a photograph, explain and develop possible surgical goals, and do so right before the patient's eyes. This is extremely helpful in effective communication between doctor and patient. The goals of one patient may be very different from another. One of the integral parts of my practice is making sure each procedure is a fully unique event. I am not creating the same nose for everyone; I am partnering with my patient to create a customized surgical plan that honors your ethnicity and unique characteristics.

Although a well-executed rhinoplasty can create significant and sometimes even dramatic cosmetic improvement for most patients, there is a definite limit to how much the nose can be safely altered. There are anatomic considerations, such as skin thickness, skeletal size, and available blood supply, as well as functional limitations and long-term durability issues that may limit the extent of cosmetic change. Although you may want a specific look—for example, an ultra-slender nose like Paris Hilton's—rhinoplasty can seldom transform a nose from one extreme to another, and attempting to do so could lead to complications.

That said, any healthy patient could have a well-proportioned nose with elegant lines and a more pleasing contour thanks to rhinoplasty.

Ideal Candidates for Rhinoplasty

The best candidates for rhinoplasty are those looking for improvement, not perfection. They are well-adjusted folks, otherwise happy with their lives, and do not expect rhinoplasty to transform them into someone else.

How do I assess if my patients meet these criteria? I listen carefully and attentively. I ask non-judgmental questions to establish a rapport based on trust, encouraging them to be honest and open with me so I can better understand and, ultimately, better meet their goals and expectations for the surgery.

Too Young or Too Old for Rhinoplasty?

There are certain age-related factors that should be taken into account when considering rhinoplasty. It is best to have a patient wait until after any "growth spurts," as nasal growth can destroy the proportions that were made during surgery and create an unbalanced nose. The nose is usually fully developed between the ages of fifteen and seventeen for boys and fourteen and fifteen for girls. Also, younger children may not be ready to face the emotional trauma of cosmetic surgery, so each case needs to be reviewed to allow the surgeon to make an accurate determination.

For adults in good physical and mental health, age is not a factor. In fact, rhinoplasty for those in their thirties, forties, and fifties is relatively common. Rhinoplasty, in conjunction with other procedures such as a facelift or eyelid surgery, can make a dramatic difference in how vital and youthful a person appears.

The belief that the nose never stops growing is only partly true. As the body ages, the nose does indeed lengthen slightly and look more prominent. The tip of the nose drops and elongates, so by the time a person reaches the age of fifty or sixty, that might appear in some people as a "bump."

In actuality, the nose did not develop a bump, but the relative position of the dorsum (external ridge of the nose) as compared to a "dropped tip" gives the appearance of a bump.

Also, the stretching and lengthening of the "smile muscle," which is used countless times over a lifetime, can further deteriorate the overall look of the nose. Rhinoplasty can restore a more youthful look and prevent some future drooping.

In both adults and young people, reconstructive rhinoplasty can be used to repair previous nasal injury or obstruction brought about by physical trauma or to correct the results of a previous procedure.

The Difference between Men and Women

Rhinoplasty is different for men and women in many respects. Facial aesthetics, or what surgeons call "ideal aesthetic standards," differ between the sexes, especially when it comes to the nasolabial angle— the angle between the nose and the upper lip, as seen in the side-view profile on the following page.

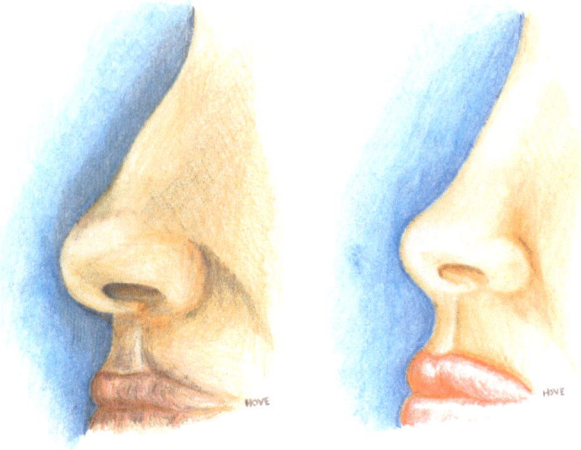

Typically, the more ideal standard for a male is a smaller angle, about 90 degrees, while for a woman, it is a little more opened up, about 100 to 105 degrees. This is based largely on average male and female heights, as you don't want to look at someone's nostrils. The shorter the individual, the more you want to have that angle a little more open.

Another consideration is the thickness of the skin, as it plays an important role in the results of the operation. Thick skin will not "drape out" as well over the new underlying structure. However, thicker skin can hide small irregularities of the cartilage and bone better than very thin skin.

Although most people are eligible for rhinoplasty, there are times when a surgeon will advise against the procedure. It is important that you disclose all existing medical problems or list any medications you are taking, as certain conditions may make it unsafe to undergo rhinoplasty. Also, if a surgeon believes a person's reasons for seeking surgery are "unhealthy"—for instance, they involve underlying emotional issues or unrealistic expectations—the doctor has the right and even the obligation to refuse to perform the rhinoplasty.

Chapter 3

The Rhinoplasty Procedure

As a surgeon I can make your nose larger, shorter, smaller, straighter, or thinner by recontouring the underlying cartilage and bone of the nose. The tip of the nose, for example, can be corrected by adding or removing cartilage at the tip and stitching the cartilage together. On the other hand, a low tip of the nose can be raised by adding cartilage to support the tip, removing excess cartilage in the septum, or repositioning the cartilage.

Rhinoplasty can also correct:

1. The dorsal bone by removing excess cartilage and bone to lower the height;

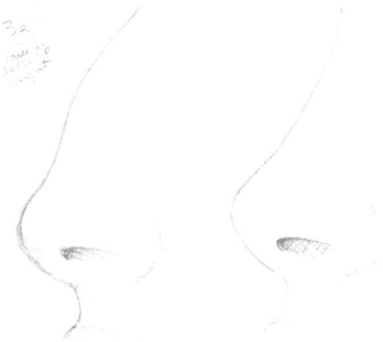

The sketch on the left demonstrates a bump or dorsal convexity. By lowering the dorsal height, the nose is left to look more feminine and/or aesthetically more pleasing.

2. The wide, bony portion of the nose with a controlled fracture of the nose and repositioning it inward;

3. The wide or flared nostrils of the nose, by removing tissue at the base of the nose, moving nostrils closer together;

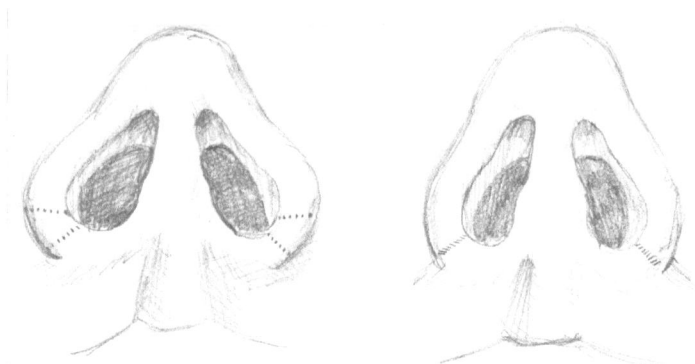

4. The angle between nose and lip, which creates the illusion of a droopy tip, by modifying the septum.

The sketch on the left illustrates what is described as a droopy or ptotic tip. Correction of this can be performed during rhinoplasty, leaving the patient with a more aesthetically pleasing profile.

Rhinoplasty Surgical Choices: Open vs. Closed

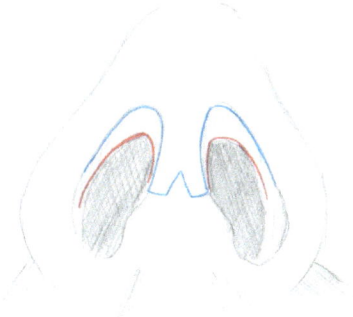

The different incisions used for rhinoplasty are shown here. The red incision is an incision made on the inside of the nose, or more commonly referred to as the closed approach. The blue incision is made somewhat more external and is associated with the open approach.

There are two techniques used in rhinoplasty surgery—open rhinoplasty and closed rhinoplasty. In open rhinoplasty, the surgeon carefully makes an incision in the *columella*, the fleshy column of the nose sandwiched between the two nostrils. The nasal skin is then lifted back to expose the underlying cartilage and nasal tissue. Additional incisions are placed inside the nose. The incision placed outside usually heals well and, if well executed and sutured carefully, rarely causes cosmetic problems. These incisions are not straight lines but usually some form of a zigzag to make them less noticeable.

The closed or *endonasal* rhinoplasty surgery is performed through access incisions in the inside of the nose. I personally prefer to perform a closed rhinoplasty. It leaves no visible scarring since incisions are made on the inside of the nose and, as a result, patients have less bruising, swelling, and discomfort after the operation. This also shortens the postoperative healing and recovery time, which minimizes downtime—one of the primary concerns of rhinoplasty patients.

In the last 20 years there has been a huge increase in popularity for the open approach and especially among younger, less experienced surgeons. Their argument is that the open approach allows them to better visualize the anatomy leading to a more predictable result.

On the other hand, experienced rhinoplasty surgeons who advocate for a "closed" or endonasal approach argue that it is a much less invasive approach. (I subscribe to this thinking.) They also believe that with experience, the results are as predictable, or even more predictable than the open approach because of the less invasive nature of that surgery. There are new studies supporting this position.

However, the endonasal procedure requires exceptional surgical expertise and artistic insight. A highly skilled surgeon can use the closed procedure for most rhinoplasty operations. That said, there are certain indications when a surgeon, including myself, will prefer the open for extensive nose surgeries.

When deciding on open vs. closed rhinoplasty, talk with a reputable and experienced rhinoplasty surgeon. Since open rhinoplasty is the preferred procedure for most surgical residents in training, providing a greater opportunity for observation, many new surgeons have developed a greater expertise in the open rather than closed procedure. The closed rhinoplasty requires more experience, specific training, and, frankly, a keen interest in learning this procedure. For this reason, when choosing a surgeon, be sure to ask which procedure he or she prefers, why he or she prefers this particular method, how often he or she performs it, and why it is *or is not* the best method for your circumstances.

Where to Have Your Rhinoplasty Surgery

I've chosen to operate in my own accredited ambulatory surgery center. I believe this is the optimal situation for my patients since I have all the essential backup systems and the same safety standards as a hospital. We have all the rigors and standards of a federally inspected hospital *without* any unnecessary exposure to germs and illnesses.

While a surgeon can also get his or her office accredited to accommodate an operating room, an accredited ambulatory surgery center operates at a much higher standard. In my center, for example, we have climate-controlled air exchanges, which comply with hospital standards. In short, our operating rooms are identical to those in a hospital; we're just not attached to one.

Also, the same team works with the patient throughout the surgical procedure and postoperative period, rather than sharing a recovery room with multiple patients, and our patients receive one-on-one, dedicated care, customized for the aesthetic surgery patient. We have the ability to transfer patients to the hospital. In my fourteen years of performing surgery in our own surgery center, I haven't had to use this option, but it is there. I do have patients to whom I recommend a hospital setting for their rhinoplasty due to certain medical conditions.

Another advantage of the accredited ambulatory surgery center is lower surgical fees for the patient. There are no extra layers of bureaucracy, so we're able to pass those savings on to the patient.

The Initial Consultation with Your Surgeon

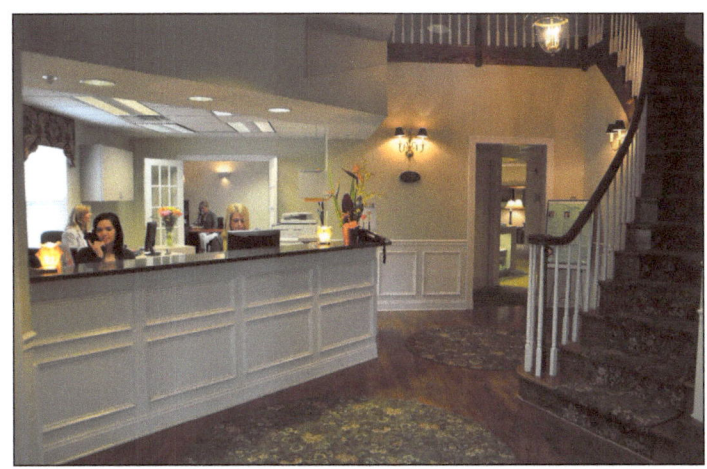

Should you opt to go forward, your next step is to select a highly regarded, experienced surgeon. This is, without a doubt, the most important part of the process. To start, consider doing a web search, or ask a trusted doctor or rhinoplasty patient for a referral.

Board certification, in my opinion, is a minimum standard. It does not, however, constitute training in a specialized area. The average plastic surgeon finishes his or her training having completed no more than four or five rhinoplasties. It is strongly recommended that you choose a surgeon who has dedicated his or her primary practice to this particular procedure.

Ask any surgeon you are considering if rhinoplasty is a major focus of his or her practice. If the surgeon and/or the staff can look you in the eye and say *yes* without batting an eye, you are most likely dealing with a doctor highly skilled and experienced in rhinoplasty.

The more focused on rhinoplasty a surgeon's practice, the more referrals he receives from his colleagues and the more often he is performing the operation. As a result, their skills are sharp and well-honed. They are often educating others on a national or even international level and are considered a leader in the field. This is the level of competency and care you want for your rhinoplasty.

Once you schedule an appointment, consider what information you would like to know about the surgery and the doctor performing it.

Don't be reluctant to ask for the surgeon's credentials or rhinoplasty experience. Feel free to bring photos and magazine clippings of noses that appeal to you. Obviously, a nose that looks beautiful on someone else may not suit your face; however, it may help your surgeon visualize what you want.

A confident and competent surgeon will appreciate this opportunity to assure you and put you at ease. It's also a wonderful way to build rapport, facilitate greater communication, and increase the likelihood that your expectations will be understood and met.

Depending on where you live, there may not be a thriving local practice or very many to choose from, but don't let that get in your way. Consider the option of traveling to the best surgical practice for an initial consultation, which, in most instances, will be worth the additional time and relatively modest fee of about $150.

Once you arrive at the office you will be given paperwork to fill out prior to your preconsult with the doctor's staff. You may also have the option, as in my practice, to download and print out necessary patient information forms from the practice's website, complete them ahead of time, and bring them to your appointment.

These include:

New Patient Information Form

New Patient Medical History Form

HIPAA Contract*

HIPAA Notice of Privacy Practice*

Preop Anesthesia Form

Patient Medicine Reconciliation Form

Postop Instructions for Nasal Plastic Surgery

---

* These forms explain your rights under HIPAA—the United States Health Insurance Portability and Accountability Act of 1996—regarding how your medical information may be used and disclosed and how you can get access to this information.

Take a Look Around

While you wait to meet with the surgeon, take a look around the office. Does it exude competence and caring? Do you feel at ease? Is the waiting room clean and comfortable? Is the staff courteous and professional? Are there articles about the doctor, videos from local and national media, certificates of board approval, professional journal articles, or perhaps thank-you cards from previous patients that assure you are in a first-class practice?

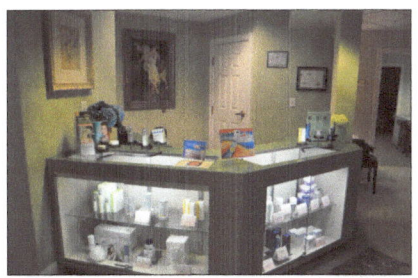
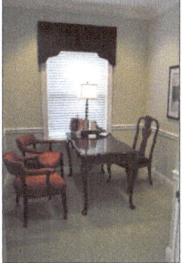
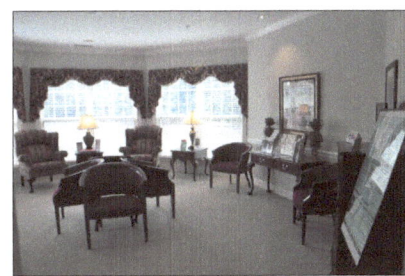
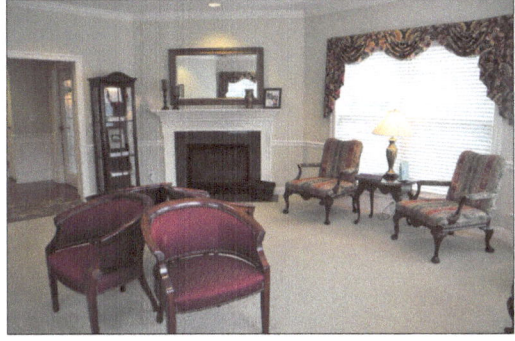
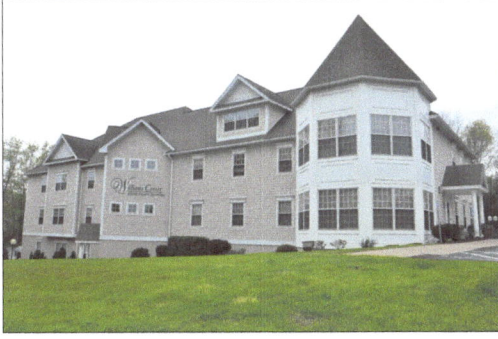

It's not just about décor, environmental aesthetics or first impressions. Such efforts demonstrate the physician's commitment to provide you and all his or her patients with the best possible experience.

Rhinoplasty Consultation Checklist

I have included a helpful **Rhinoplasty Consultation Checklist** to take with you to your consultation. Although a good surgeon will cover all the necessary points, it is best to have a written list so nothing important is missed—especially as you may be understandably nervous during the consultation.

RHINOPLASTY CONSULTATION CHECKLIST

As you consider the best surgeon for your rhinoplasty, there are important questions you want the surgeon or his staff to answer. The Consultation Checklist below includes such questions and provides an easy way to remember them as well as keep track of a surgeon's responses.

Plastic Surgeon's Name:

Office Phone Number:

Date of Consultation:

Time of Appointment:

Credentials

Are you Board Certified?	Yes	No
American Board of Facial Plastic and Reconstructive Surgery?	Yes	No
American Board of Plastic Surgery?	Yes	No
American Board of Otolaryngology—Head and Neck Surgery	Yes	No

Additional board certifications: _____

Rhinoplasty Experience

How long have you been performing rhinoplasty?

How many rhinoplasty procedures have you performed?

How many times do you perform rhinoplasty in an average year?

Do you perform open rhinoplasty or closed rhinoplasty? Both?

Do you teach other surgeons rhinoplasty surgery?

Have you been published on the subject of rhinoplasty?

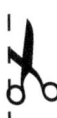

Surgical Procedures

Ask to see before and after photos of some of the doctor's rhinoplasty patients.

Can I speak with one of your past rhinoplasty patients?   Yes   No

Where will the surgery be performed? _____

Is the surgical facility an accredited ambulatory surgery center? Yes   No

If yes, by whom? _____

Feel free to ask for a tour of the surgery facilities.

At which hospital(s) do you have admitting privilege/s?

_____

Medical Conditions and Medications

Write down any of your existing medical conditions to discuss them with the plastic surgeon. Also make a list of the medications you are taking, and don't forget to include vitamins and other supplements, as they can cause interactions with anesthesia or other medications. I have included the **Medications, Vitamins, and Supplements to Avoid List** on page 35 to help with this process.

Rhinoplasty Costs

What is the cost for the surgery?

Does this include the costs of anesthesia, surgical facilities, etc.? Yes   No

If not, what are the additional costs?

Do I need to buy any medications before or after the surgery?   Yes   No

What kind of pain medications will I be given?_____

_____

What are they and what might they cost?

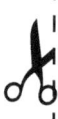

Do I need to buy medical supplies (ice packs, nasal sprays, etc.)? Yes   No

If so, what will they cost? _____

Who can I talk to about my payment options, including insurance coverage and financing? _____

Anesthesia

What type of anesthesia will you use? _____

Who will administer the anesthesia? _____

What are their credentials? _____

The Rhinoplasty Procedure

Describe the procedure and provide any imaging or diagrams that will help me understand it.
_____

How do you remember what was discussed during my consultation?
_____

What complications can occur?
_____

Postoperative Care

Are there any special instructions I should follow once I get home?

Are they available online?_____

What should I be on the alert for after surgery that might indicate a need to call you?_____

What is the rhinoplasty healing process like? _____
_____

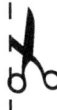

A CGI Is Worth a Thousand Words

You may be reluctant to have a rhinoplasty because you're afraid the shape of your nose after surgery will not be what you expected or wanted. Computer-generated imagery (CGI) can help alleviate such fears, as it gives you and your surgeon a visual idea of what your nose will look like after surgery.

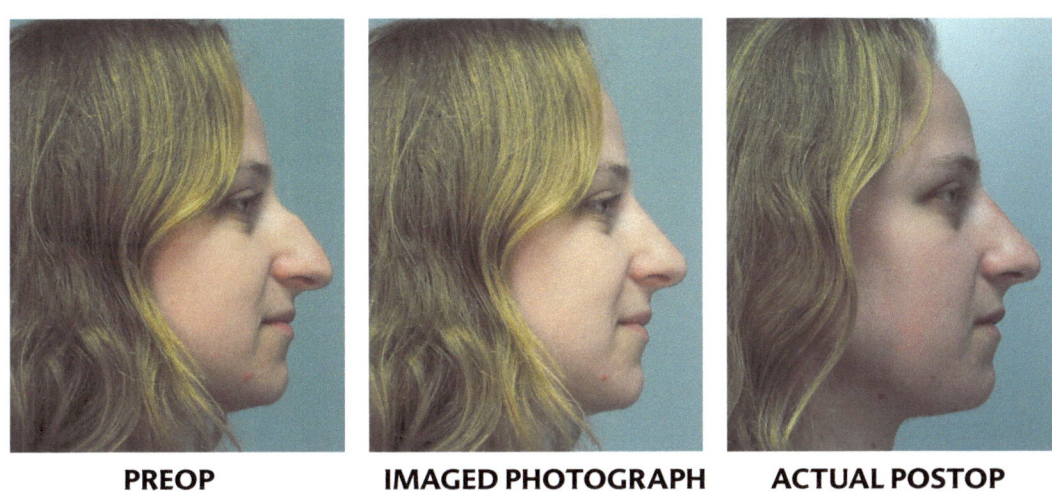

PREOP   **IMAGED PHOTOGRAPH**   **ACTUAL POSTOP**

That's why computer imaging is an essential part of my practice, as it allows patients to communicate their aesthetic wishes in visual form. At the same time, it gives me the opportunity to display what sort of results I feel are achievable and realistic given the patient's nasal anatomy and skin type. There is no guarantee your new nose will exactly match the one shown to you in the simulation, but it can help you feel more confident in proceeding with surgery.

How exactly does CGI work? At the time of your visit, photos are taken and put on the imager, a computer with a screen for viewing. These images usually take about fifteen to twenty minutes to create, and I save them to use as a guide during surgery. The images are not a guarantee of results but rather a visual representation of our mutual surgical goals for your nose. Computer imaging gives you greater assurance that the surgeon is shaping your nose the way you want it.

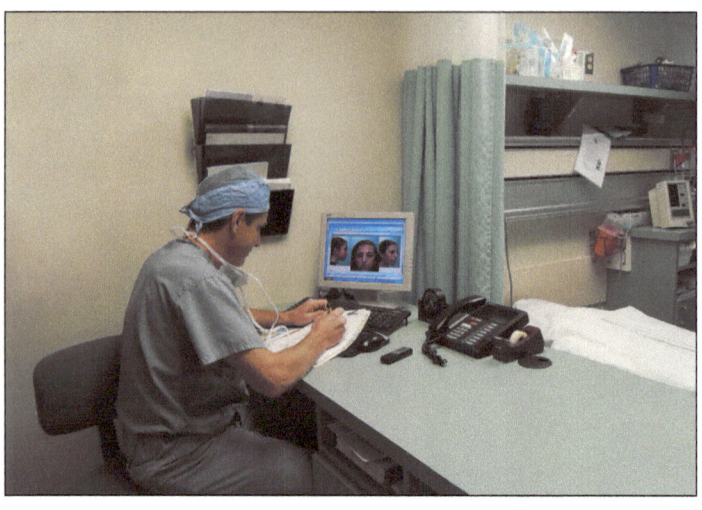

You will be given a consent form for the CGI. Be sure to read this carefully so you fully understand all the points listed on it.

During the consultation, with the aid of imaging, diagrams, and hand sketches, the surgeon will give you a comprehensive overview of the rhinoplasty procedure and discuss your options, such as where you would prefer the incisions to be placed. Most surgeons have a portfolio of before and after pictures of their rhinoplasty operations that demonstrate their skill and expertise. These pictures can help you and your surgeon "get on the same page" about what's possible in cases similar to yours. A good practice can also arrange for you to speak with patients to discuss their experience with the practice and the surgery as you decide whether or not to go forward.

I've noticed that some patients worry that I may forget the particulars of their case, given the span of time between their consultation and the date of surgery may be several weeks apart. For this reason, I let them know during our preoperative appointment that I take very detailed notes, thoroughly review imaging photos, and then design a specific plan for their surgery.

At the end of the consultation, you will meet with the surgeon's staff to review fees, costs, and payment options. If you are certain rhinoplasty is for you and you have chosen the right surgeon, you can schedule your surgery along with preop requirements such as an EKG or physical examination. Remember, you are not obligated to commit to the surgery at the end of the initial consulting. If you need more time to think over your decision, by all means take it. You owe it to yourself to consider any reservations. You will not be the first or last person who comes to such a decision after a consultation.

The key to a successful consultation is thorough preparation. Good communication between you and your surgeon will increase the likelihood of getting the nose you want. Speak up and take an active role in the consult and in the process that follows.

Chapter 4

Before Your Rhinoplasty (Preoperative Preparation)

At your preoperative appointment, your doctor's staff will give you instructions to follow before and after your rhinoplasty surgery. These should include when to schedule your next appointment, prescriptions for antibiotics, swelling and pain medications, and recommended supplements for faster healing.

Some surgeons recommend taking vitamin C (ascorbic acid) as well as Arnica, a natural herb, two weeks before and after surgery, as they can decrease bruising. It's best to obtain all prescriptions and medications before your surgery so they are ready when you return home.

Again, be sure to let your doctor know about your daily medications (bring a list for easy recall or use the one on page ___ as a guide) so he or she can let you know which of these can be taken (with just a sip of water) the morning of your surgery and which must be avoided. For example, medications including aspirin or ibuprofen should be avoided two weeks before the surgery. If you are taking prescription blood thinners, such as Coumadin and Plavix, do not stop taking them without a discussion with the prescribing physician. Include any vitamins, herbal supplements, or diet pills, as they may contain elements that thin the blood and interfere with anesthesia.

Increase fluids a few days prior to surgery. We find that patients recover faster from anesthesia when they are well hydrated, and we encourage them to increase their water intake a few days before surgery.

Just remember—do not eat or drink any food or liquids after midnight the day before the surgery, including water, candy, mints, or gum. You can brush your teeth.

The night before surgery, feel free to wash your hair and face. Don't apply makeup on the morning of the surgery. Leave all jewelry at home including rings, earrings, watches, and any piercings. Contact lenses should not be worn the day of the surgery. Eyeglasses are acceptable and can be brought into the operating room with you.

You'll want to wear comfortable clothing, such as yoga or sweatpants and a shirt or sweater with front closures to avoid pulling it over your head and risk hitting your nose after surgery.

I prefer to perform rhinoplasty with a combination of general and local anesthesia. In the local mixture, there is a small concentration of epinephrine, which constricts blood vessels and helps reduce bleeding. You will not feel the injection of local anesthesia, as it is administered while you are already sedated.

Your surgeon might give you a choice regarding anesthesia, depending on your particular circumstances. If you have any concerns, don't hesitate to ask him or her why he or she is recommending a particular anesthesia.

Medications, Vitamins, and Supplements to Avoid

Aspirin and aspirin-related products should not be taken two weeks before or after surgery because they increase the tendency of bleeding. For this reason, it is very important that contents of any over-the-counter preparations be checked carefully prior to their use. Many headache preparations, cold remedies, and "hangover cures" contain aspirin. The chemical name of aspirin is acetylsalicylic acid.

Examples of drugs containing Aspirin (acetylsalicylic acid):

Acetidine	Coricidin	Excedrin	Midol	Robassisal
Alka-Seltzer	Cephalgesic	Feldene	Mobidin	Roxiprin
Amigesic	Cheracol Caps	Fenoprin	Monogesic	Rufin
Anacin	Clinoril	Fiorinol	Nabumetone	Saleto
Anahist	Congesprin	Froben	Nalfon	Salflex
Anaprox	Children's ASA	Flurbiprofen	Norgesic	Sine Off
Anaproxin	Choline Salicylate	Gelprin	Norwich EX	Sine Aid
Ansaid	Cope	Genpril	Ocufen	SomaCompound
APC	Corticosteroids	Genprin	Orudis	Suldinac
Argesic	Coumadin	Goody's Body	Oruvail	Synalgos DC
Arthra G	Daypro	Haltran	Oxyphenbutazone	Tanacetum
Arthropan	Depakote	Halfprin	Oxybuta	Trandate
Ascodeen	Dilofenac	Ibuprin	Oxyprozin	Trigesic
Ascriptin	Dipyridamole	Ketoprofen	Pamprin	Trental
Aspergum	Disalcid	Ketorolac	Peptol Bismol	Trilisate
Aspirin	Divalproex	Lortab ASA	Pecodan	Tusal
Baby Aspirin	Doan's Pill	Liquiprin	Persantin	Vanquish
Bayer	Dolobid	Magan	Phenaphen	Voltaren
BC Powder	Dristan	MG Sallicylate	Piroxicam	Warfarin
Bromo-Quinine	Easprin	Meclofenamate	Ponstel	WillowBark
Bromo-Selzter	Ecotrin	Meclofen	Prednisone	Zactrin
Brufen	Emprazil	Medipren	Quagesic	
Bufferin	Empirin	Mefenamic	Relafen	
Butazolidin	Endodan	Menadob	Rexolate	

Examples of aspirin-related products (Ibuprofen, Indomethacin, Naproxen, Tolmetin)

Advil	Naprosyn	Indocin	Tolectin
Aleeve	Nuprin	Motrin	Toradol

You can substitute *Tylenol occasionally* for the products above; however, avoid taking it *daily* for two weeks prior to surgery.

If you are taking regular prescription medications for high blood pressure, diabetes, heart disease, or asthma, *PLEASE check with your doctor before surgery before disrupting your routinely scheduled medications.*

Supplements:

It is important to discontinue the use of the following supplements two weeks prior to surgery, and for up to two weeks after surgery:
- Bilberry ▪ Cayenne ▪ CoQ10 ▪ Dong Quai ▪ Echinacea ▪ Feverfew ▪ Fish Oil Caps ▪ Garlic ▪ Ginger ▪ Ginseng ▪ Ginkgo Biloba ▪ Hawthorne ▪ Kava Kava ▪ Licorice Root ▪ Ma Huang (ephedra) ▪ Melatonin ▪ Red Clover ▪ Valerian ▪ St. John's Wort ▪ Vitamin E ▪ Yohimbe ▪ Multivitamins

ALCOHOL—Abstain from any drinking two weeks prior to and after surgery. Alcohol can cause postoperative bleeding and delay healing.

NICOTINE—Nicotine interferes with healing by reducing blood flow. Avoid smoking, as well as gums and patches which contain nicotine, for at least two weeks prior to your procedure.

Risks and Complications of Anesthesia

Anesthesia is very safe, especially when administered by an anesthesiologist or nurse-anesthetist. But safe does not mean there is no risk. You need to understand what the risks are and tell your surgeon if you have any heart or respiratory problems. Other underlying problems, such as liver or kidney disease, can interfere with anesthesia and raise the chance of an adverse event. Smokers are more likely to have problems with anesthesia than people who do not smoke.

Remember, thousands of people have anesthesia safely every day. Most of the associated risks are very small and unlikely to happen. The vast majority of people undergoing surgery with any type of anesthesia do just fine.

This information is not meant to alarm you but rather to inform you so you can make a well-educated decision about your anesthesia.

Fasting before Surgery

Your stomach needs to be empty in the event you become nauseated during or immediately after your surgery. This means no breath mints, lozenges, or gum. If you must take a medication the morning of your surgery, consult with your surgeon *first*. It is important to follow your surgeon's preoperative instructions to avoid any problems.

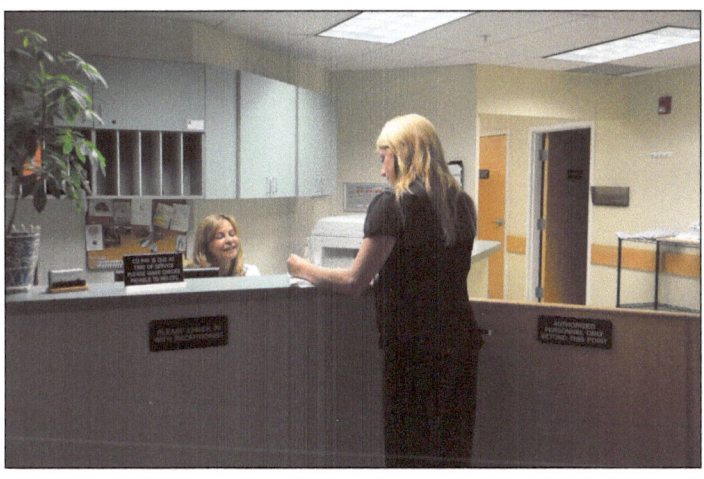

The Day of Your Surgery

When you arrive on the day of your surgery, you will review and sign consent forms and answer some important questions regarding whether you have any allergies to medications, or have had anything to eat or drink since the night before.

The nursing staff, anesthesia provider, and other health professionals will ask these questions several times before your surgery—this is for your safety and protection. The open and frequent exchange of information helps ensure a safe and successful procedure.

During this time, I like to check in one more time with my patients to address any concerns or questions they may have.

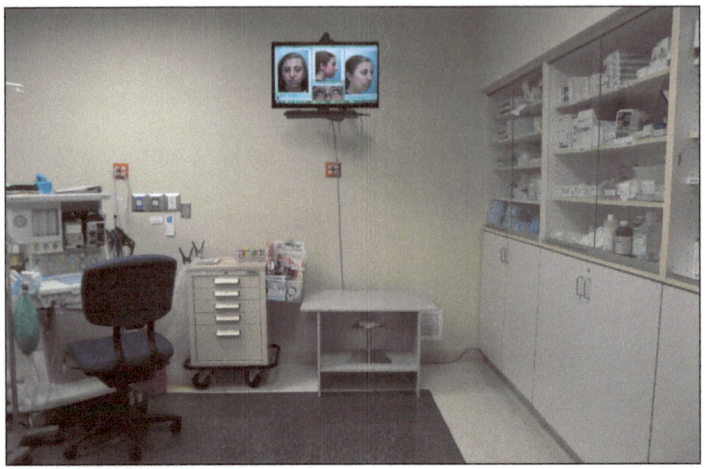

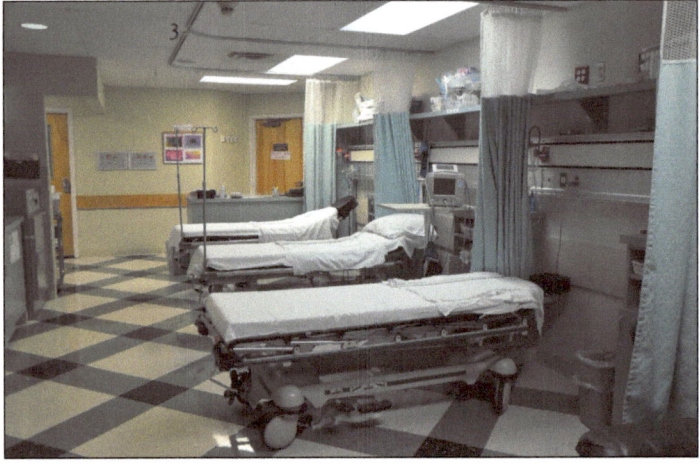

I also let my patients know their photos and images will be displayed on the monitors in the operating room. These help me refer to the subtler aspects of their nose, which may be less obvious during the procedure due to swelling from local anesthesia and from the patient laying flat on the table.

Next, a nurse or other health professional will start an IV with fluids that contain antibiotics as well. Once you are in the operating room, you will be given sedation so you will be asleep and quite comfortable during the procedure.

Rhinoplasty takes about an hour and a half, depending on the structure of the nose and the extent of the changes made. (If you are having a combination of procedures, your surgery will take longer.)

During this time you will be pain free, relaxed, and kept still thanks to anesthesia, which is administered by a certified registered nurse-anesthetist (CRNA), or an anesthesiologist (a medical doctor who specializes in anesthesia).

You will awaken from anesthesia with an external drip pad or "mustache dressing" taped to your upper lip to catch any drainage. There may be internal nasal dressings as well, especially if a septoplasty (to straighten the nasal septum, the partition between the two nasal cavities) was performed.

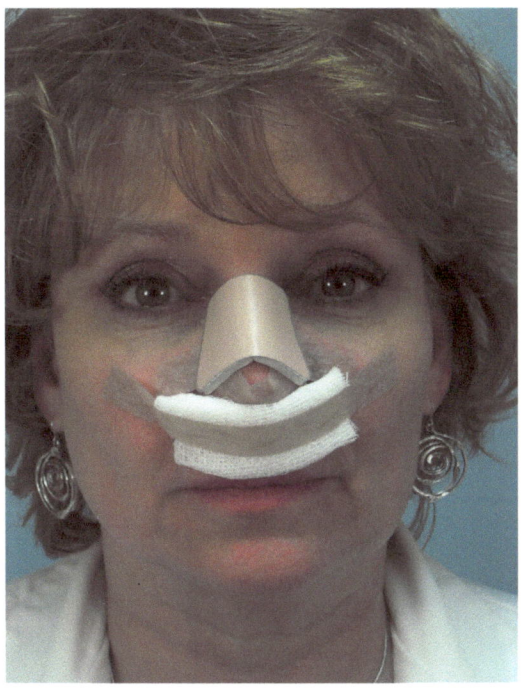

The rhinoplasty nasal splint remains in place for a week after surgery.

Your nose will be in a metallic splint like the ones used to set a broken finger. These are much cleaner and more contemporary than messy casts.

Some surgeons still *pack the nose* by applying gauze or cotton packs to the nasal chambers. The most common purpose of nasal packing is to control bleeding following surgery to the septum or nasal reconstruction or to provide support to the septum after surgery.

I've found this unnecessary in holding the nose or the septum in position, as the nose should be where you want it to be when the surgery is done. I have also found it's the packing that makes many patients extremely uncomfortable, especially as it inhibits their breathing.

Instead of packing the nose, I use a light, soft dressing made of Telfa, which feels like the gauze side of a Band-Aid. A small piece is folded in half and slipped in each nostril to catch the drainage, which will subside in a short time. *If you are completely saturating the drip pad with bright red blood every five minutes for an hour, notify your doctor. This can routinely be treated with instructions over the telephone or with an office visit.*

Your mucous membranes might produce extra mucous, some of it red tinged, and may leak through this light dressing onto your drip pad. This is normal. Ice packs to the forehead and/or back of the neck may help decrease bleeding, but avoid placing ice packs directly on your nose splint. Also, be sure to cough up and spit out any drainage from your nose, as swallowing it may make you sick to your stomach.

Use a lozenge, such as Cepacol, if your throat is sore or mouth is dry from the anesthesia after surgery. Drinking as much fluid as possible will prevent dehydration. Keep your favorite drinks handy—water is best—and consider a humidifier (cool or warm) for added comfort. Use Vaseline, ChapStick, or lipstick to moisten your lips.

You may also notice that tears run down your cheeks. This is due to swelling and will subside during the first week following rhinoplasty surgery. The dressing removal will also help relieve some of the pressure that you may feel.

Chapter 5

After Your Rhinoplasty (Postoperative Procedures)

In my practice, patients are given instructions to remove the dressing inside the nose the day after surgery. Most patients describe the removal as a relief of pressure rather than painful. I encourage my patients to take their pain medication about an hour prior to removing the packing to take the edge off any discomfort.

Some patients prefer to have the doctor or his staff remove the dressing. In my practice, we are happy to do this for you during a routine office visit.

Once the dressing (inside the nose) is removed, you will breathe easier; however, don't blow your nose just yet.

The splint must remain on your nose for one week after your rhinoplasty surgery. It must be kept dry or it could become loose. Notify your facial plastic surgeon immediately if the splint falls off.

I know people can be anxious about having the splint removed. They'll say, "Is it going to hurt?" No, it does not hurt, and if you get in the shower about an hour before your appointment and get the splint wet, it softens and is then easier to remove. Once the splint is removed, you can clean up any remaining adhesive on your skin with little acetone (or nail polish remover).

Saline Rinsing

The evening *following* splint removal, start your saltwater rinses. Saltwater rinsing is very important for your postoperative rhinoplasty healing. The salt water moisturizes, cleanses, and facilitates healing.

You can make "homemade" salt water by mixing one tablespoon of sea salt (not table salt) and twelve to sixteen ounces of lukewarm water in a small plant mister bottle. Place the tip of the mister gently near the opening of the nose, and spray your nose. If you prefer, you can purchase saline spray at the drugstore without a prescription. Rinse your nose with salt water five to six times a day for one week. Then you can cut it back to three times a day.

Medications

You will be offered a prescription medication for swelling. Most rhinoplasty patients complain of pressure from swelling and congestion more than they do pain. Typically, my patients tell me that their pain threshold on a scale of 1 to 10 is, on average, a 2.

However, painkillers (Loritab or Vicodin) are generally prescribed for the first day or two after surgery. If your pain is mild, consider taking an extra-strength Tylenol (acetaminophen) according to manufacturer's directions instead. Do not take additional Tylenol while taking Loritab or Vicodin, as they contain acetaminophen. Do not drive or drink alcohol while taking any prescription pain medication. Side effects of pain medications can include nausea and constipation. Taking pain medication with food can minimize nausea. If you are inclined toward constipation, drink plenty of fluids and/or take a stool softener (as directed) starting the evening of surgery.

Most patients find they can switch to Tylenol after a day or two. Please check with your doctor before resuming any other medications taken on a regular basis.

As you may recall, you received IV antibiotics during your rhinoplasty surgery. You'll need to continue this protection, so start your antibiotic (Keflex or Cephalexin) when you arrive home after the procedure and take it as directed until finished. Keep in mind that it is not uncommon to have a low-grade fever for twenty-four hours following surgery.

Nasal congestion, facial fullness, headache, and disrupted sleep are also normal postoperative rhinoplasty symptoms. You may also experience some numbness on the roof of the mouth (palate) behind the front teeth, so avoid extremely hot liquids or food immediately after the initial postoperative period.

Don't worry—these will decrease as the healing process occurs.

Chapter 6

Additional Postoperative Recommendations

Rest quietly in bed (or in a reclining chair) with your head elevated (above the level of your heart) for the first forty-eight to seventy-two hours after surgery. Continue sleeping elevated for approximately one week, and, if possible, on your back for a few weeks afterward. Consider sleeping alone for a week or two after surgery to avoid someone else accidentally bumping your nose.

It is common to have low energy levels following surgery. Unnecessary activity will encourage swelling, discomfort, and bleeding. Minimize all activities for several days until these symptoms resolve. *Resist using your recovery period to catch up on errands, exercise, or home projects. You need rest.*

When you resume social activities and return to work really depends on you. The average patient returns to work or social activities in seven to fourteen days. At about two weeks, you can start with aerobic activities; however, avoid anything involving contact for three weeks. After this period, most patients are healed and can get back to contact activities knowing that any direct hit to the nose could result in additional surgery.

Ninety percent of rhinoplasty patients see little or no bruising four to five days after surgery. Most patients have only a little wisp of a bruise under each eye. This is important to note, as patients mistakenly believe they will suffer more serious bruising for as long as three weeks.

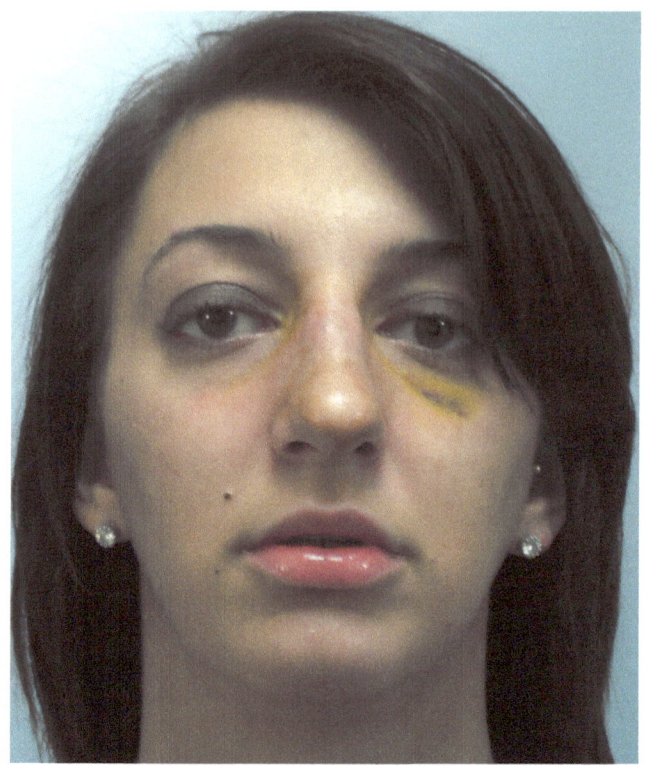

As you can see from this photograph, rhinoplasty leaves some bruising.

At my practice, we discovered using a pulsed dye laser a week or so after surgery is very effective in minimizing or eliminating bruises. This is rarely necessary with rhinoplasty. If you have concerns about your appearance during recovery, you can consult a professional makeup artist. Ask your plastic surgery practice for a recommendation.

When and What to Eat

In most cases, a healthy appetite will return within twenty-four to forty-eight hours of anesthesia. Start eating when you feel hungry. Consider light liquids (broth, soda, crackers, toast, etc.) and progress slowly to regular foods. Increase fluids such as water and fruit juices (no citrus fruits). Avoid alcohol, nicotine, and caffeine, as these will dramatically slow the healing process.

Caring for the Nose

Do not put ice on the splint.

Avoid showering or any direct spray of water on the face around the nasal splint for a week after the procedure, as the nasal splint should remain dry and in place during this time.

Do not adjust or play with the splint, tape, or dressing. (Your doctor will remove the splint approximately one week after surgery.)

Avoid bumping or hitting the nose. Notify your doctor if you experience an accidental blow to the nose causing excessive swelling and bleeding.

Avoid excessive movement of the upper lip. Do not pull the upper lip down when applying lip balm, lipstick, or gloss.

Avoid excessive grinning and smiling. (You'll have to smile on the inside for awhile.)

Avoid "sniffing" or forcibly attempting to pull air through the nose.

Avoid constantly rubbing the base of the nose and nostrils with a Kleenex or handkerchief.

Avoid sneezing. If you must sneeze, do so through your mouth.

Eyeglasses cannot be worn as long as the splint is on. They must be suspended off the bridge of the nose. This is important, as the pressure of the glasses may change the new contour of the nose. The doctor's staff can show you how to tape the glasses in such a way to avoid any problems.

No contact lenses for forty-eight hours after surgery.

Avoid sun exposure as much as possible.

First Postoperative Appointment

Your first return appointment will be approximately six to seven days following surgery. At this time, your physician will check your nose and remove the splint. We usually take a set of photos at this time for comparative purposes.

Some patients experience discouragement or mild depression after cosmetic surgery. It is natural to be concerned when your face is a bit swollen and bruised.

The Results Take Time

Remember, it takes time for the swelling of the mucus membranes to subside and for the skin to adhere to the new framework. As I've said, most patients return to work one to two weeks following rhinoplasty surgery, depending on temporary bruising and swelling. The swelling may appear very obvious to you but many of your coworkers and closest friends will not notice.

You will see 80 percent of the changes after just one week and 90 percent after two weeks. After three months, the changes are ever so subtle, although still significant. Your final result following rhinoplasty is not fully apparent for one year following surgery. This is what makes this surgery so interesting and complex. A surgeon has to have the skill and the vision to make a rhinoplasty work for his or her patients over time.

Conclusion

According to the American Academy of Facial Plastic and Reconstructive Surgery (AAFPRS), a half a million people a year, interested in improving the appearance of their noses, seek consultation with facial plastic surgeons. Like you, they may be unhappy with the nose they have or the way it is changing as they age, or they may be looking to fix an injury that has changed their nose or caused breathing difficulty. One thing is true in all cases: nothing has a greater impact on how a person looks than the size and shape of the nose, so even a slight alteration can greatly improve one's appearance.

While no book can completely address all your concerns and questions, it is my hope that this one has provided answers to many of them.

Successful facial plastic surgery requires good communication between patient and surgeon. It requires trust, based on realistic expectations and exacting medical expertise and developed in the consulting stages before surgery is performed. I encourage you to take whatever remaining concerns you have to a surgeon who can better address your specific needs.

I find this work especially rewarding—to create a nose that fits a person's face or to improve his or her breathing while positively contributing to his or her overall confidence and self-esteem—is my life's work.

It is exciting to play a role in creating tremendous, and sometimes dramatic, improvements in a patient's quality of life.

I've enjoyed sharing my expertise, knowledge, and experience with you, and, whatever you ultimately decide, I hope this book has proven to be a richly informative resource.

Chapter 7

Rhinoplasty—FAQ

Preoperative

1. **Is rhinoplasty painful?**
   Rhinoplasty is performed under anesthesia, so the procedure itself is not painful. All patients are given pain medicine for the first few days. However, most patients do not complain of significant discomfort and typically take just Tylenol the first few days. The occasional patient will feel the need to take prescription pain medications the first evening after surgery. The most common complaint by patients is the inability to breathe through their nose the first night after surgery. We put in each nostril a light Telfa dressing, which is removed by the patient the next morning, allowing the patient to breathe more freely. It is not unusual for us to be told by the patient at the first week postoperative visit that he or she had little or virtually no discomfort from his or her procedure.

2. **What is a "hanging columella"?**
   A hanging columella is the central part of the nose above the lip between the nostrils. From the side view, when this is drooping it is referred to as a hanging columella. This can be corrected during rhinoplasty to create a more balanced and youthful face.

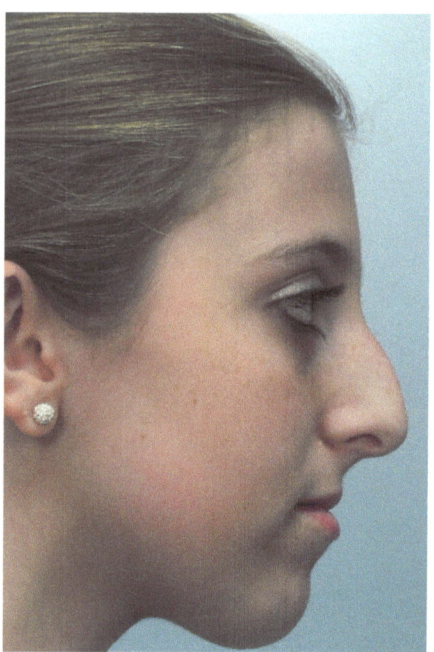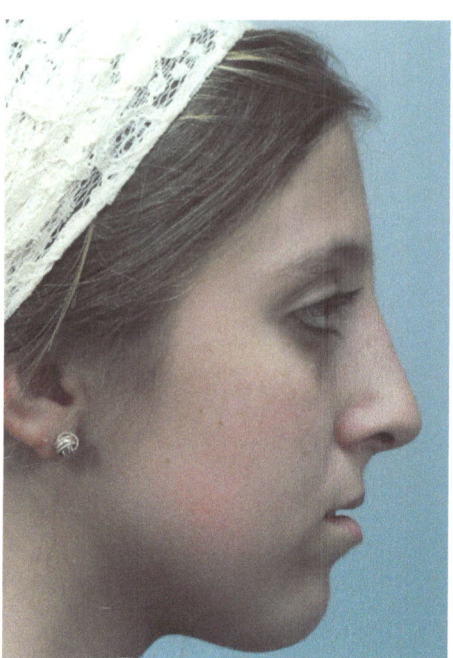

HANGING COLUMELLA CORRECTION

3. **Are there any complications or risks with rhinoplasty?**
    With all surgical procedures there are risks and potential complications. It is the surgeon's responsibility to manage risks and to discuss them with the patient. The risks I generally discuss with patients are the potential for infection or bleeding. Although it is extremely unusual for a patient to have any significant bleeding after rhinoplasty, we want to be sure we inform our patients of this possibility. If any issue with bleeding arises, it will typically happen within the first few hours and patients must return to the office to have that addressed.

4. **Can I combine cosmetic rhinoplasty with other facial surgery?**
    The short answer is yes. Many patients will have rhinoplasty performed either with another facial procedure or even a body procedure. For example, it is not unusual for patients to have rhinoplasty in conjunction with a blepharoplasty (eyelid surgery) or breast augmentation. It requires a consultation and examination by your doctor regarding the different procedures.

5. **Is it appropriate to ask to speak with my doctor's previous rhinoplasty patients?**
    Absolutely. We encourage patients to speak to someone else treated by the practice that has had a procedure similar to theirs. The more information a patient has, the better, and this is certainly an appropriate request by the patient.

6. **Will my health insurance cover my rhinoplasty?**
    A portion of rhinoplasty can be covered by health insurance in certain circumstances. Typically this will occur when a patient has a deviated nasal septum, nasal valve collapse, or a previous history of trauma or injury to the nose. In those particular circumstances, the breathing or functional component of the nasal reconstruction is covered by a patient's health insurance. If the rhinoplasty is solely for cosmetic change or improvement, it is not covered by insurance and is the patient's full financial responsibility. This should be discussed in detail at the time of the initial consultation so patients understand what portion of the cost is covered and what portion is not.

    Surgeon's fee average $7,3 00 and up depending on location and cost of living variables. This would include operating room and anesthesia fees, which are based on the amount of time needed to perform the surgery.

7. **Is it possible to get financing for rhinoplasty?**
    Yes. Most surgical practices, including mine, offer several options for financing, including health care financing plans such as Care Credit and/or a preoperative layaway approach. Depending on your circumstances, there may be additional options, so be sure to review these concerns with the surgeon's practice during your initial consultation.

8. **What if I decide to have my breathing problem fixed at the *same* time as cosmetic surgery to change the shape of my nose?**
    Changing the outside appearance of your nose is considered cosmetic, which is an out-of-pocket expense. Insurance companies will generally cover the cost of the medically necessary part, such as your breathing problem. Even with the additional expenses for the cosmetic rhinoplasty, it is important to understand you still have an obligation to the insurance company to make any copays, deductibles, etc.

9. **Do you have advice for African American persons on choosing a plastic surgeon?**
    Most highly experienced rhinoplasty surgeons are experienced in addressing all ethnic groups. Choose a surgeon with significant rhinoplasty experience, as he or she will be familiar with the subtleties of preserving ethnicity in either African American or other ethnic backgrounds.

10. **As a result of cocaine addiction, I have a hole inside my nose, between my nostrils. Can I have the hole filled?**
    Yes. What you are referring to is what is called septal perforation. It is important for the doctor to assess this, as the success rate for repairing a septal perforation is not 100 percent. Much of it depends on the size of the perforation and the location. For example, a septal perforation that is located to the front and is a certain size is amenable to being repaired. Larger septal perforations are posterior (in the back part of the nose) and have a much lower success rate. This naturally requires an evaluation by a competent surgeon who is experienced in septal perforation repair. In my practice, our success rate with septal perforation is very high because we carefully evaluate the patient's potential for a good result.

11. **What health conditions threaten a successful recovery after rhinoplasty?**
    The conditions that threaten a successful rhinoplasty concern the inner structure of the nose, but these are rare. For example, someone who has Wegner granulomatosis (WG), a condition of the cartilage of the nose, in my opinion would be contraindicated for surgery. We would not perform rhinoplasty because the complication rate would be high, and we value the health of our patients. Other than WG, there are very few medical conditions that would threaten a successful recovery.

12. **How much time passes between the initial consultation and rhinoplasty?**
    This varies depending on the patient. Most patients will have a consultation and schedule rhinoplasty between one to four months from the consultation. Many of our out-of-town patients will schedule the consultation and the surgery close together to minimize travel and take advantage of our location (which is close to the airport and within walking distance of quality lodging and accommodations). However, it is not uncommon for patients to schedule rhinoplasty six to eight months after their consultation. This is never a problem, as good-quality photographs

and detailed notes by the doctor make it very easy to accurately recall and capture the agreed outcomes for the surgery. In my practice we briefly review the surgical plan with the patient in the preoperative room to assure them we remember all the details that were discussed during the consultation.

13. Where are the incisions made?

We prefer to do the majority of our rhinoplasty using an endonasal approach. An endonasal approach means that the incisions are made on the inside of the nose. We believe this helps with the recovery period and is more along the lines of what's acceptable with minimally invasive surgical correction. In certain situations, however, an incision must be made along the base of the nose. It is perfectly acceptable to use this incision, and there are many surgeons who prefer the external incision. Again, we feel that if this can be avoided, it's certainly a potential benefit to the patient. On rare occasions, patients with flaring nostrils will need an incision at the base of the nostril, and we always discuss this with the patient beforehand.

14. Does rhinoplasty leave scars?

Anytime an incision is made through the skin, it leaves a scar. Most patients think of a "scar" as being something that is unsightly. However, surgical incisions that leave a scar are done in a more controlled fashion so that they are typically very difficult to see. Again, using the external approach, there is an incision or scar that is made along the base of the nose. Since we perform most of our rhinoplasty through the closed, or endonasal, approach, all incisions are made on the inside of the nose. Occasionally there are patients for whom we do use an external approach in the procedure or make an incision on the outside, and in those particular cases this is discussed ahead of time.

15. Are there alternatives to rhinoplasty?

There are a few alternatives to rhinoplasty, but they are limited. There are some patients who are candidates for having temporary soft tissue fillers such as hyaluronic acids, including Restylane, Perlane, and Juvederm or Radiesse, which are injected in the nose to address imbalance or contour irregularities. Again, these are somewhat limited as they can only address one specific feature of the nose.

16. **Is it true that the nose runs more after rhinoplasty?**

    No. For the first week or so, this may be, but I have never had a patient with this complaint.

17. **Will smoking affect my recovery after rhinoplasty?**

    Not necessarily. In many surgical procedures, smoking does effect the recovery period. However, when rhinoplasty is performed through a closed, or endonasal, approach it does not compromise the skin healing as much as when the open, or external, approach is used. Naturally, we discourage patients from smoking any chance we get, but it does not adversely affect the recovery period in endonasal rhinoplasty.

18. **Is it true that homeopathic remedies such as Arnica, Montana, and Bromelain can reduce swelling and bruising?**

    There is no scientific evidence to prove that these homeopathic remedies are beneficial, however we do encourage patients to use them if they are so inclined. We have seen anecdotal evidence that such remedies minimize bruising and speed healing. SinEcch™ (sinn' ekk) offers an Arnica Montana and vitamin formula designed specifically for surgery (http://www.alpinepharm.com/). The most effective way to minimize bruising and swelling is to have a very experienced, skilled surgeon with a gentle technique and efficiency. We believe this is the most important part of controlling the trauma and recovery associated with rhinoplasty.

19. **What kind of material is used when grafts are needed to rebuild the nose?**

    In our practice the primary graft is the patient's own cartilage. The nasal septum is the ideal place to get septal cartilage, and this is done at the time of the rhinoplasty. However, there are patients who require additional cartilage grafting, and in such cases cartilage is harvested from the non-structural area of the ear, or from rib cartilage when larger amounts of cartilage are needed. Rib cartilage has the advantage of being in abundant supply with great structural integrity.

20. **Am I asleep during the rhinoplasty surgery?**

    Yes. Rhinoplasty is performed under general anesthesia as an outpatient. Typically the surgery takes approximately one to two hours.

21. **Can I eat breakfast the morning of surgery? How soon afterward can I eat?**

    No. As with all surgical procedures, patients should not eat anything after midnight the night prior to rhinoplasty. Approximately one hour after a patient awakes, he or she is able to drink or eat in the recovery area.

22. **Can I go home immediately following my rhinoplasty?**

    Yes. The patients stay in our recovery area for approximately one hour before being discharged with a responsible adult to drive them home.

23. **Will I be able to drive myself home after my rhinoplasty procedure?**

    No, as rhinoplasty does require anesthesia. Typically we encourage patients not to drive for at least twenty-four hours so that the anesthesia is cleared from their system.

24. **Will I need to have someone help me out at home after my surgery?**

    Not really. We encourage patients to have someone home with them the evening of the surgical procedure in the event the doctor needs to be called. For example, if someone is feeling sick to his or her stomach, it is better to have someone else place the phone call and speak to the doctor so that the patient can be cared for appropriately.

25. **When are the stitches removed after rhinoplasty surgery?**

    Almost all the rhinoplasties we perform are accomplished through an endonasal approach. Using the endonasal approach, all sutures are placed on the inside of the nose and are dissolvable, so they do not require removal. In the rare cases where we use the open approach, or external rhinoplasty, very small sutures are placed at the base of the nose and are removed approximately one week after surgery.

26. **Is it possible for someone to be allergic to dissolvable stitches?**

    It is possible, but not likely. More commonly, dissolvable sutures can cause some irritation. Allergic reactions are rare but, in this case, the dissolvable sutures are removed rather than left to dissolve during the postoperative period.

27. Will I be given a shot of cortisone to help with some of the scar tissue in my nose?

Not usually. On rare occasions we will inject a very small amount of cortisone in the area above the tip of the nose, especially in patients who have very thick skin or excessive swelling. Surgeons who perform open rhinoplasty, where there is more swelling, are more likely to give patients a shot of cortisone in the area above the nose tip to help with swelling.

28. How many follow-up visits are needed after rhinoplasty?

We like to see patients at one week, one month, three months, and, finally, at one year.

29. When are the splints removed after rhinoplasty surgery?

We place a light metallic splint on the outside of the nose, and it is removed approximately one week after surgery.

30. When can I blow my nose?

We encourage patients not to blow their nose for the first week after rhinoplasty. After this time, we allow patients to lightly irrigate their nose with saline solution spray and start to gently blow their nose. This will help clear out the crusting and congestion over the next several weeks, allowing the patients to breathe more freely.

31. Is it okay to wear glasses after rhinoplasty surgery?

Yes. Sometimes it is difficult to position the glasses high enough on the face to prevent any pressure on the nose, so many patients will use a piece of tape to fix the glasses to the forehead, above the splint. The doctor's staff can show you how to do this for the early postoperative period.

32. When is it okay to run or lift weights?

A few days after rhinoplasty, a patient can resume walking. Lifting weights or vigorous activity should be deferred for two weeks. We allow patients to resume all physical activity, including contact sports, at approximately three weeks. It is important to realize that while the bones are mended and healed at three weeks, one can still break one's nose if hit hard enough. This should certainly be taken into consideration if you enjoy contact sports.

33. Is it possible for the nose to grow after rhinoplasty surgery?

The nose will not grow at all after rhinoplasty is performed in adult patients. With younger patients, however, the nose continues to grow, and for this reason we encourage patients to wait until girls are at least fourteen years of age and boys approximately fifteen to sixteen years of age. Typically this occurs after the second growth spurt, and at that time it is permissible for the patient to have rhinoplasty.

34. Is it true it takes a whole year before you can see the results of rhinoplasty?

Yes. While most swelling is gone after the first month, there is a slow and continuous "shrink wrap" that continues for the first year. It's just the nature of the way the nose heals. I inform patients that approximately 80 percent of the results of rhinoplasty are seen at one week, 90 percent at two weeks, and the last 10 percent of the changes occur over the next year. That's why we like to see patients for up to a year, as there are many subtle changes that occur before the final outcome.

35. What if you're unhappy with the results of your rhinoplasty?

The best way to have happy patients is to have honest, open, and effective communication during the consultation. Most skilled, reputable surgeons work very hard to manage expectations and give the patient a realistic and accurate idea of the achievable outcome. For patients that are not happy, it is important that they communicate with the doctor in the postoperative period. Many times patients are not entirely happy when the tip of the nose is still a little full or the bridge is still a little high in the early postoperative period. This is handled by reassurance and in follow-up with serial photographs to show the patient the progress that is being achieved over the first year with regard to subtle changes.

When the patient has an area of settling or irregularity (and this does occur on occasion), there are many simple procedures a surgeon can do to correct this in the early or late postoperative period. These are typically performed in the office, and, on the very rare occasion where healing has occurred unfavorably, we offer the patient a revision procedure. It is our policy to fully care for our patients, and we have never charged a patient for either a minor or more significant correction.

Chapter 8

Rhinoplasty
Before and After Photos

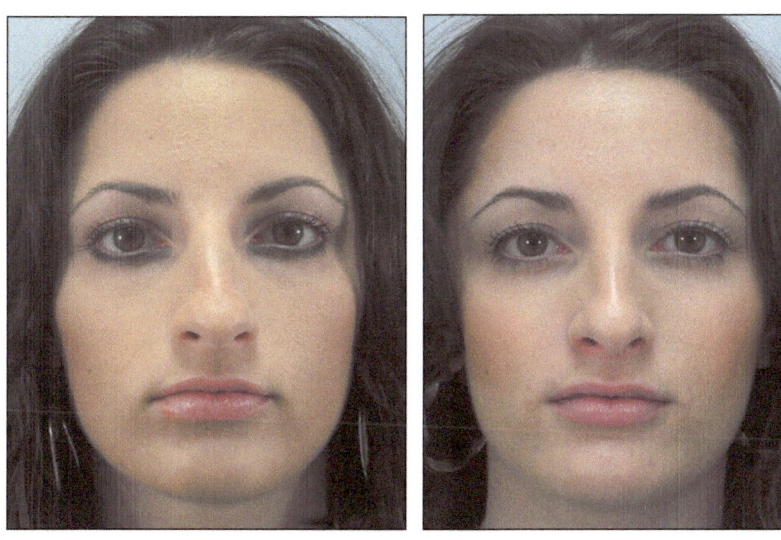

Before　　　　*After*

WIDE TIP AND BUMP REDUCED

This patient was concerned with her wide nasal tip and dorsal bump, seen here in the front and side views before surgery. The patient wanted a subtle, conservative improvement to retain her ethnic appearance.

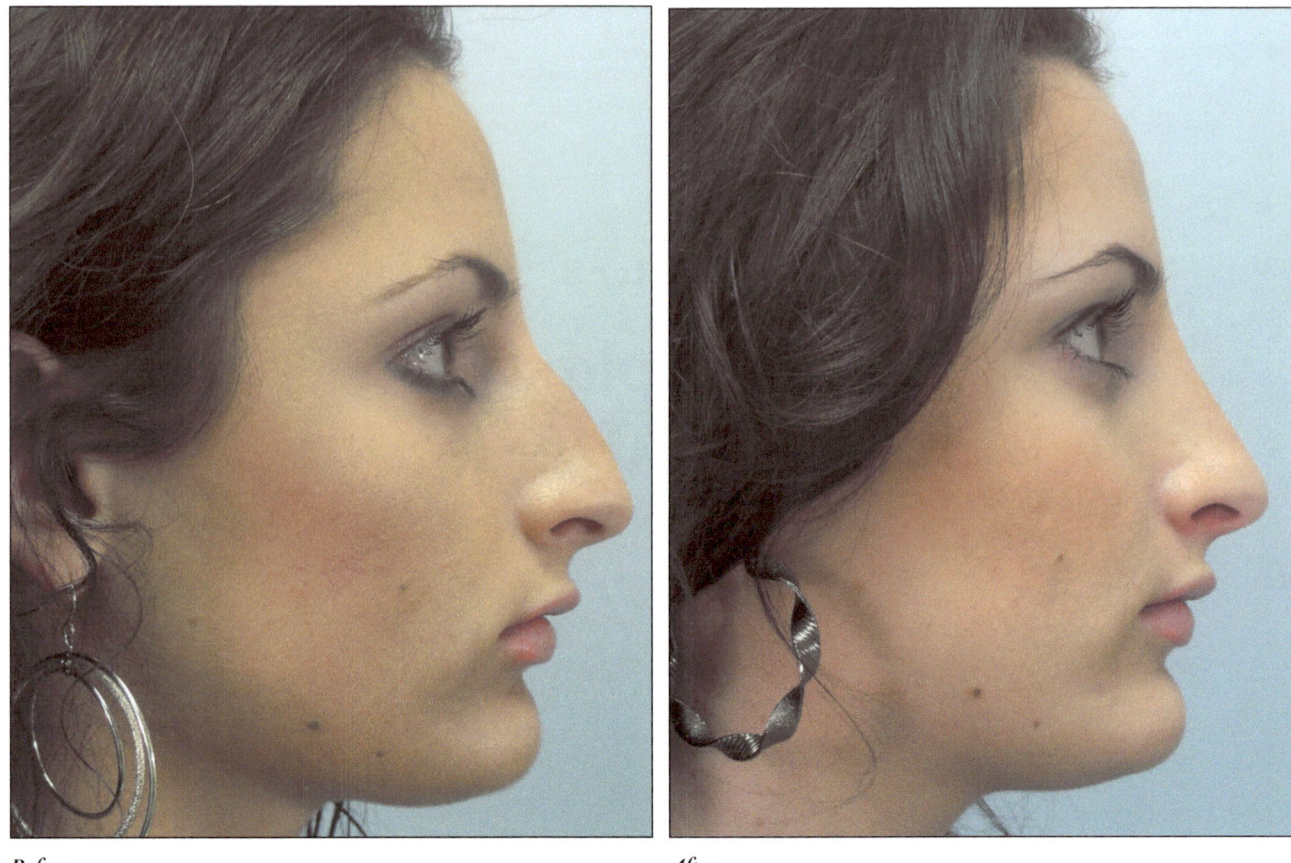

Before   *After*

WIDE TIP AND BUMP REDUCED

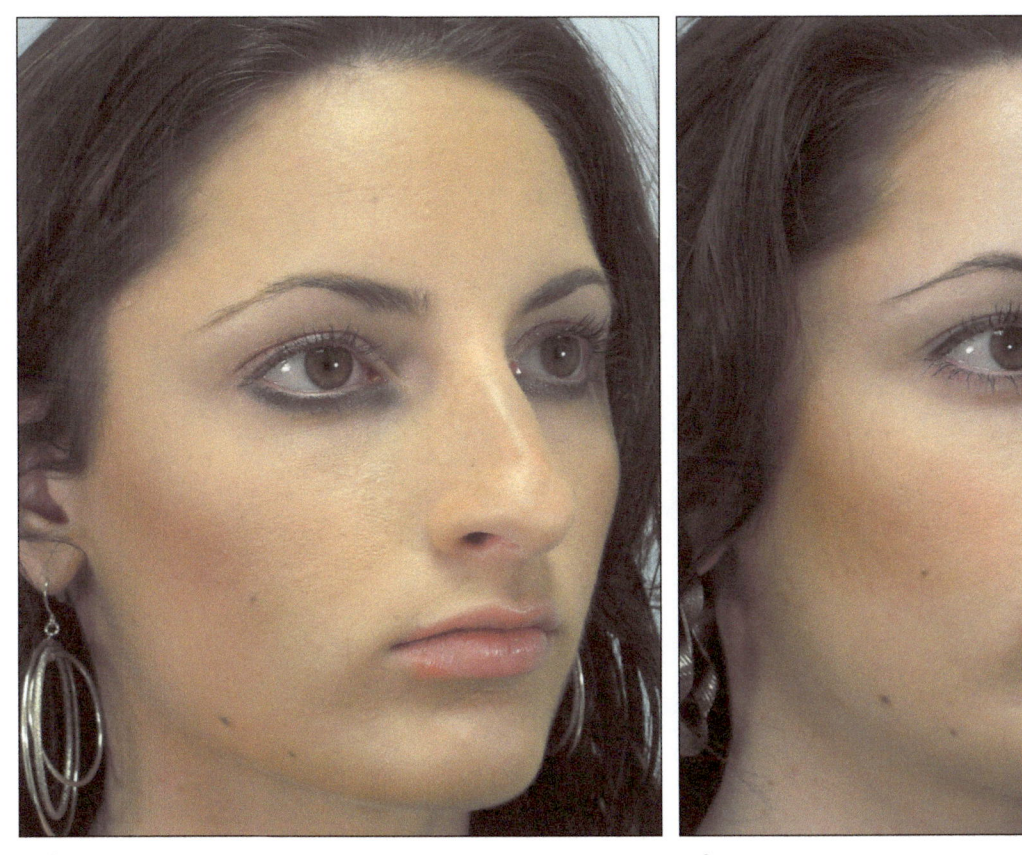

Before   *After*

WIDE TIP AND BUMP REDUCED

As you can see from her postsurgical photos, there is more refinement in the area of her nasal tip, giving her a strong yet more feminine, natural-looking profile.

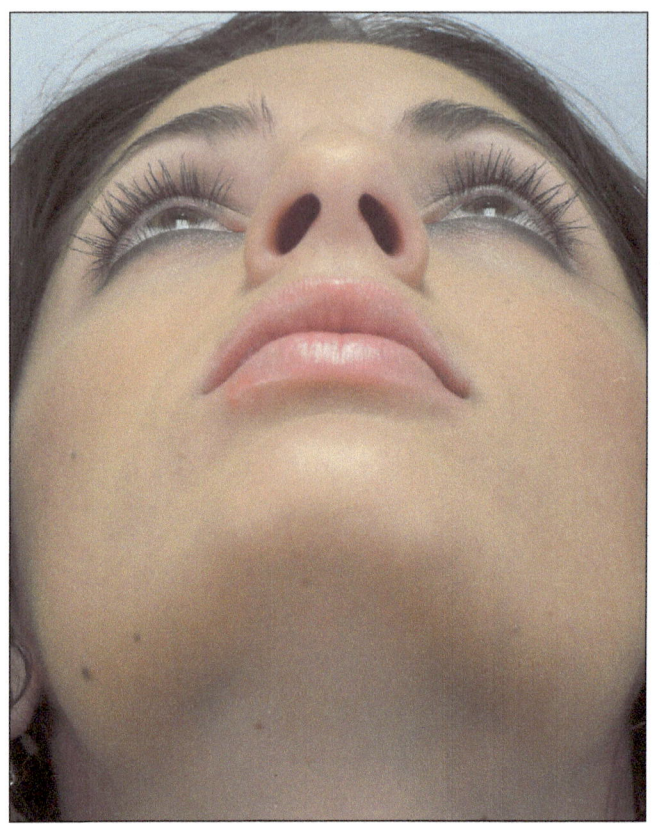

Before

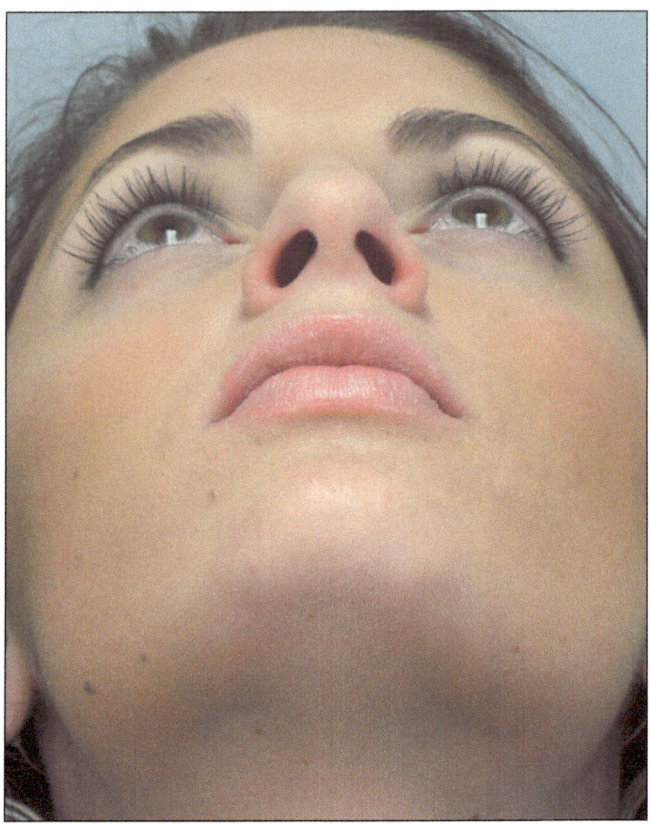

After

WIDE TIP AND BUMP REDUCED

 http://www.youtube.com/watch?v=w-KOFIDiYHs&list=PL4CDA45694188ABB0&index=5

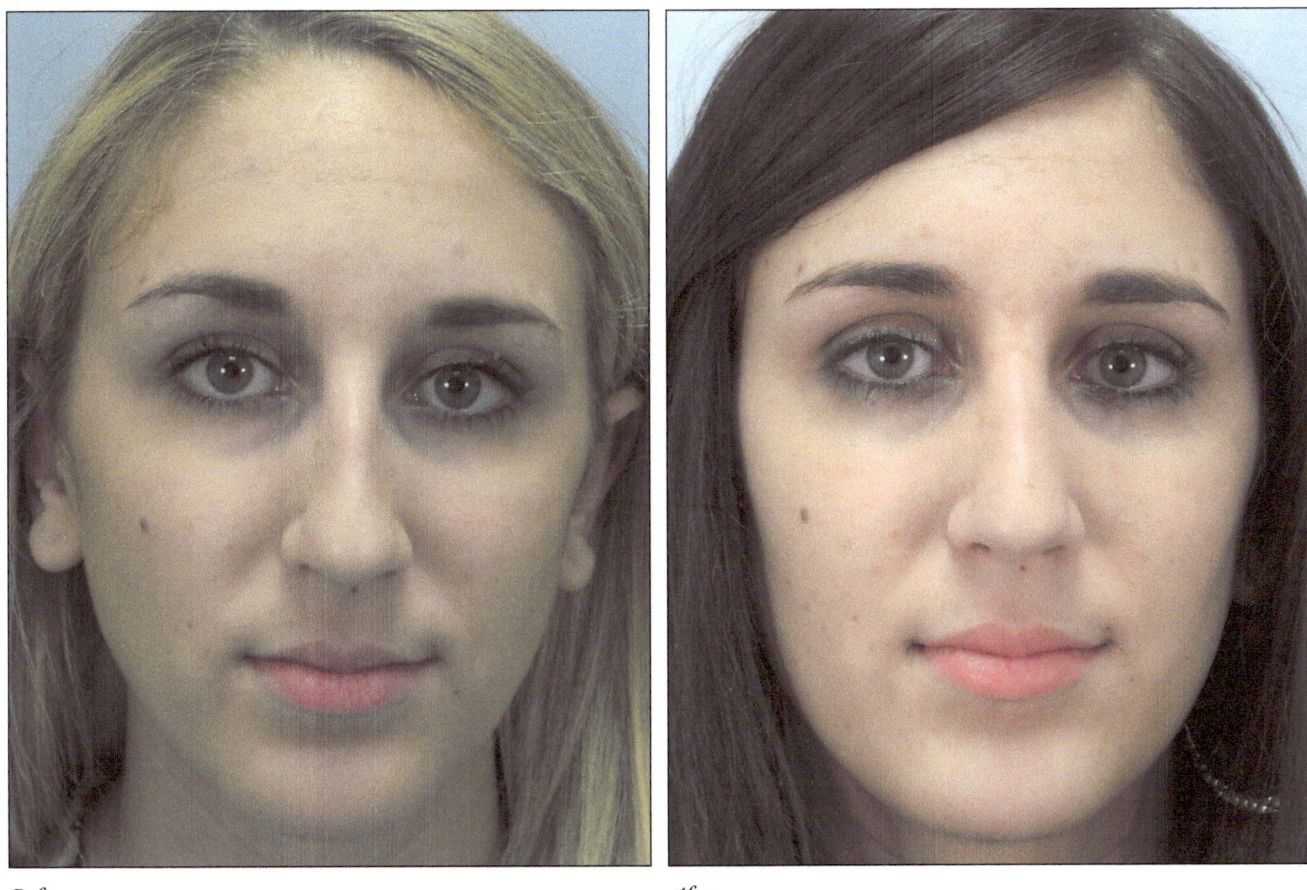

Before   *After*

NARROW MIDDLE THIRD OF THE NOSE WITH BULBOUS TIP AND DORSAL BUMP

This patient's nose is quite narrow in the middle and more bulbous at the tip. She was also concerned with the bump on her nose as seen on the following page.

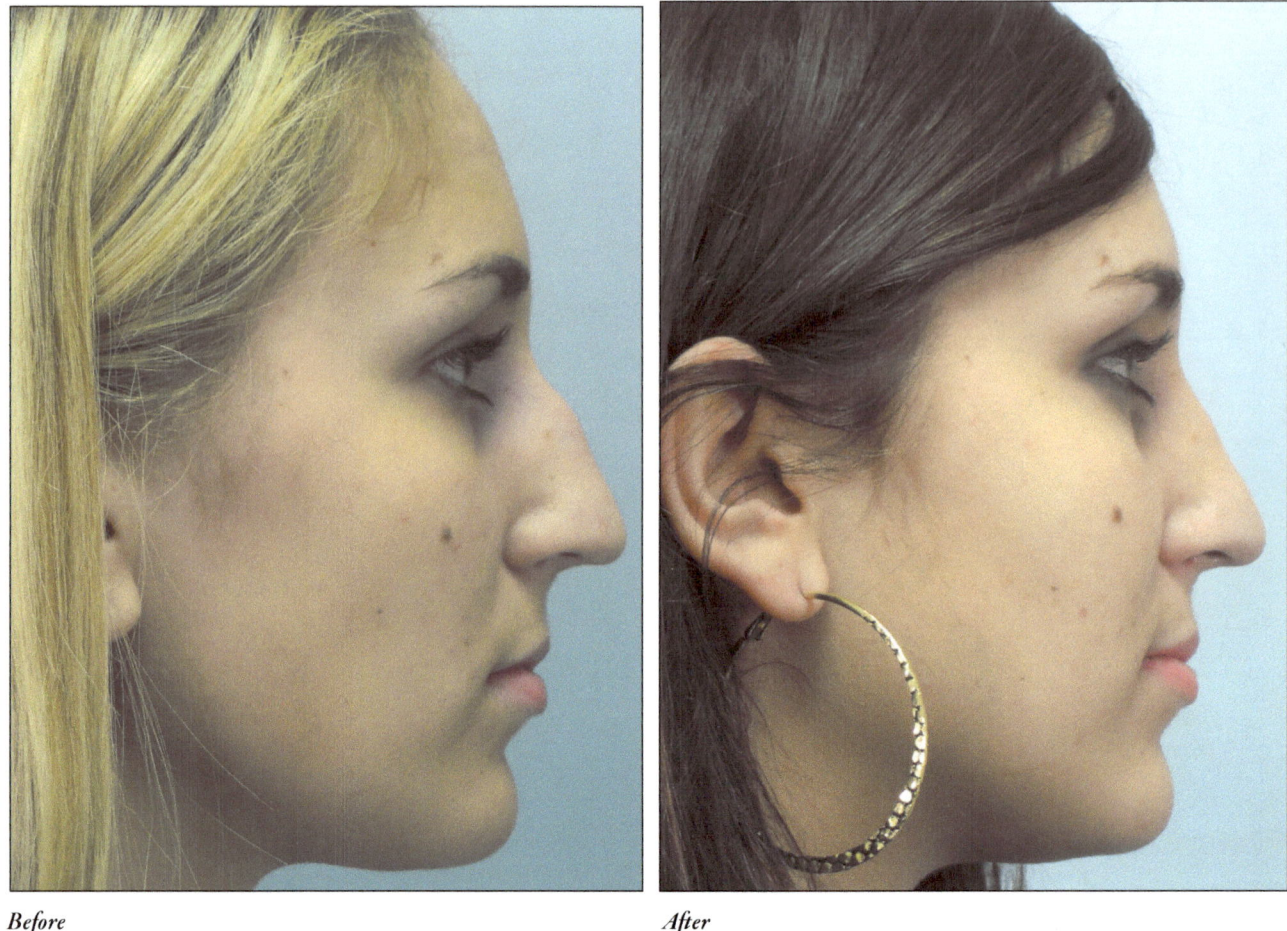

Before

After

NARROW MIDDLE THIRD OF THE NOSE WITH BULBOUS TIP AND DORSAL BUMP

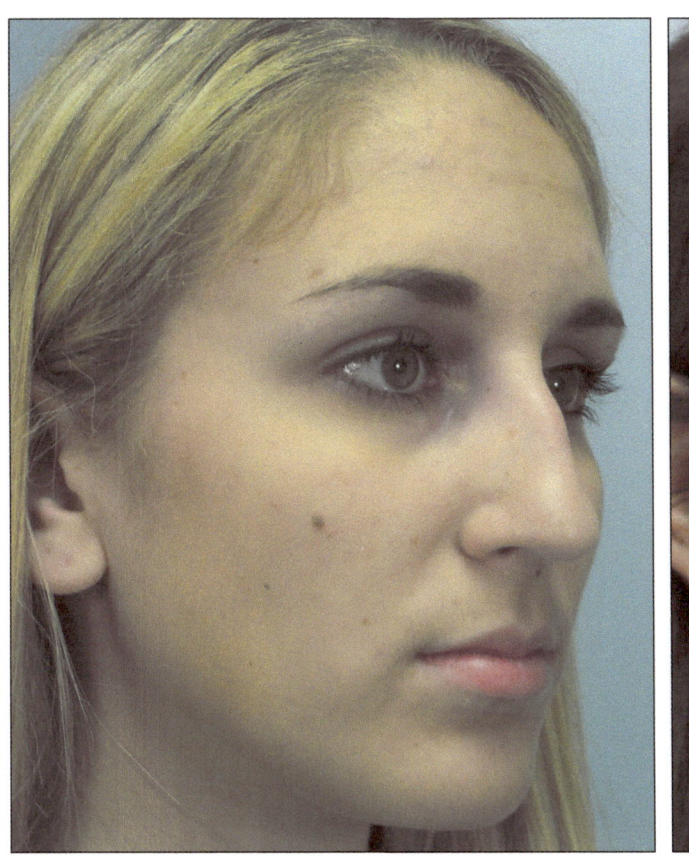

Before

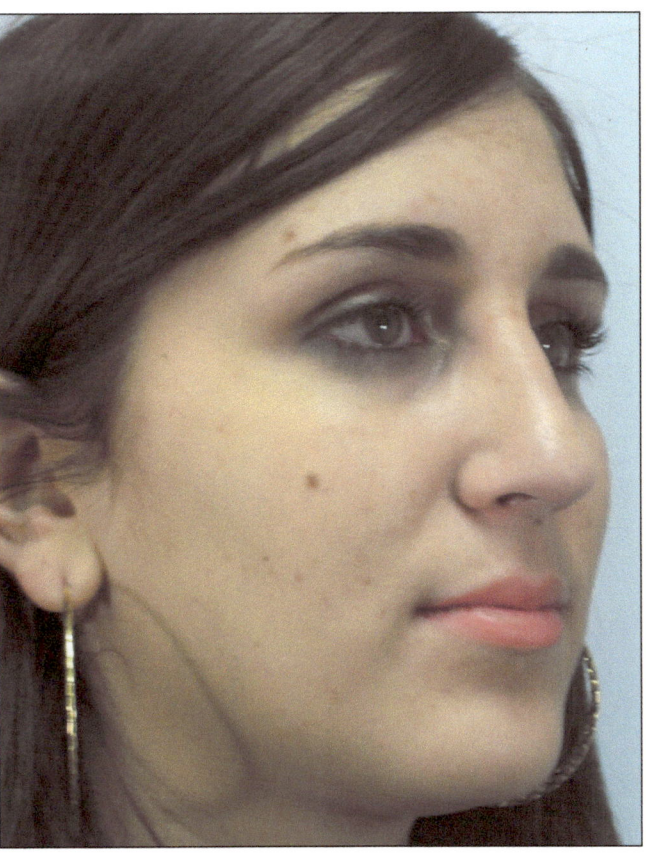

After

NARROW MIDDLE THIRD OF THE NOSE WITH BULBOUS TIP AND DORSAL BUMP

After a conservative rhinoplasty, she now has a more appealing width, improving both her middle nasal vault (middle third of the nose) and airways. Also note that the tip of the nose has been slightly rotated (approximately five degrees), which gives her nose a less droopy appearance (see previous page).

http://www.youtube.com/watch?v=M-Qo_05Gl8U&list=PL4CDA45694188ABB0&index=3

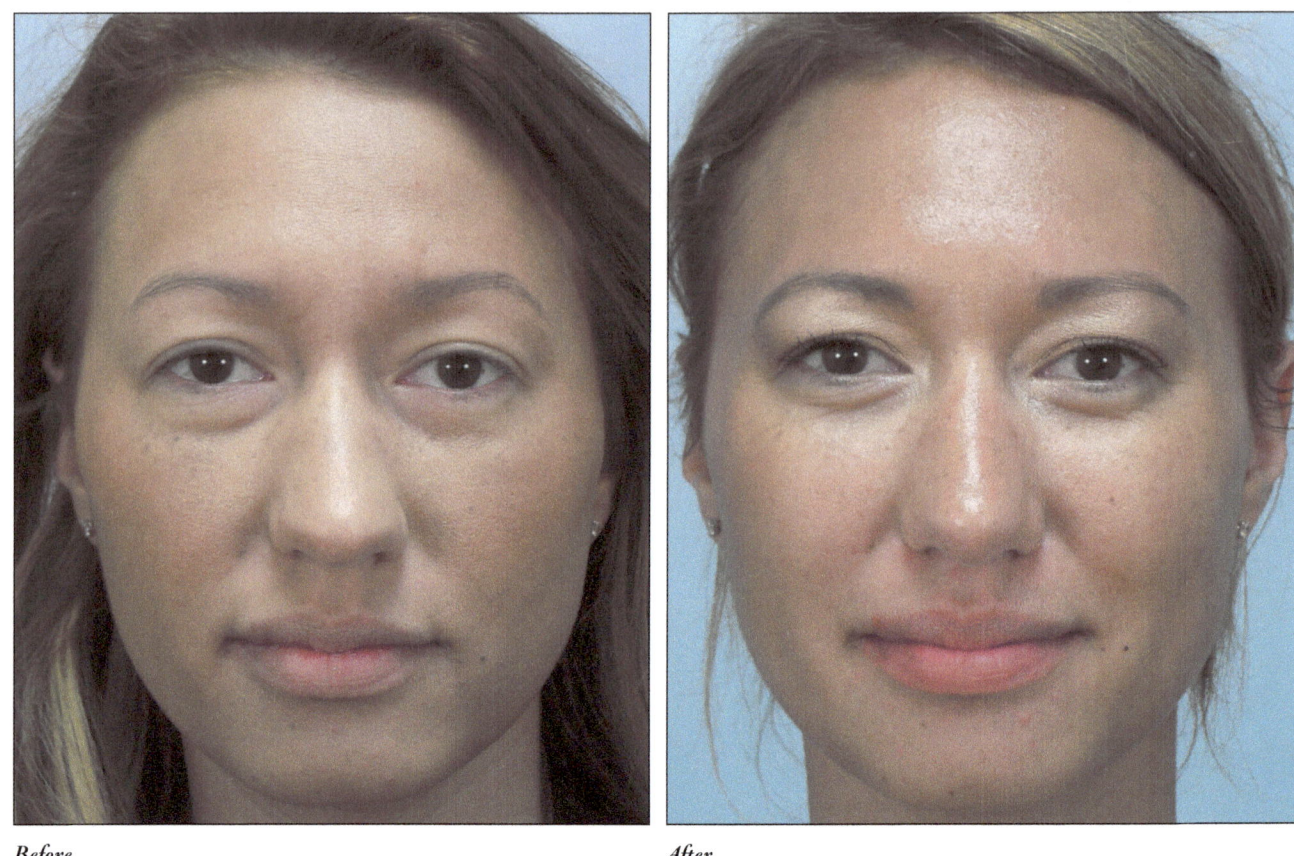

Before *After*

THICK SKIN OF THE NOSE, WIDE, DROOPY, SLIGHTLY OVER PROJECTED NASAL TIP

This patient had a slightly narrow nasal vault with thicker skin and a droopy, slightly over projected tip. In this case, an attempt to overly narrow a nose on a patient with very thick skin could leave them with a weak framework, vulnerable to some collapse, and ultimately causing breathing problems. With this in mind, during rhinoplasty the middle of this patient's nose has been widened slightly, and the tip of the nose has been narrowed as seen here and on the following pages.

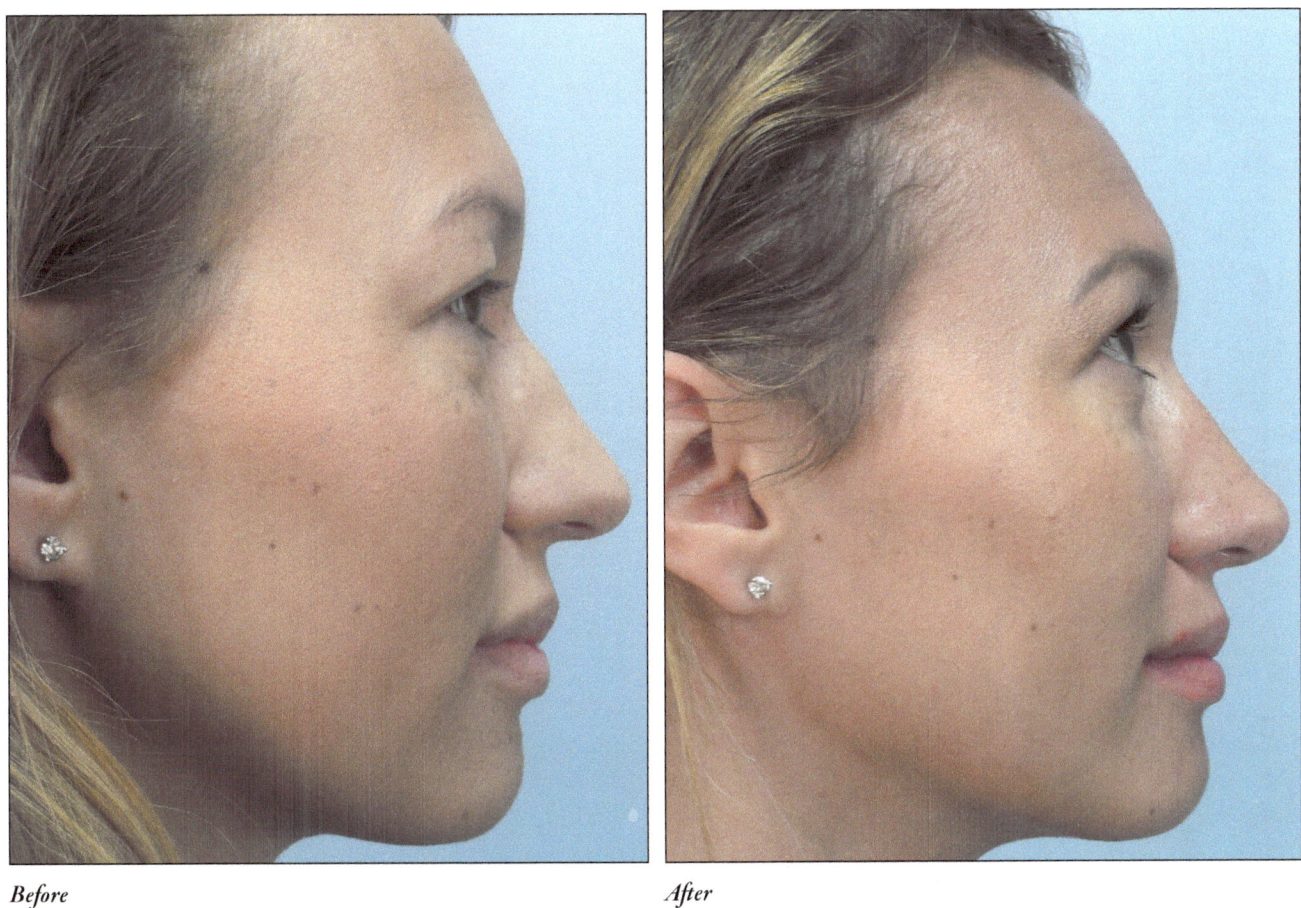

Before   *After*

THICK SKIN OF THE NOSE, WIDE, DROOPY, SLIGHTLY OVER PROJECTED NASAL TIP

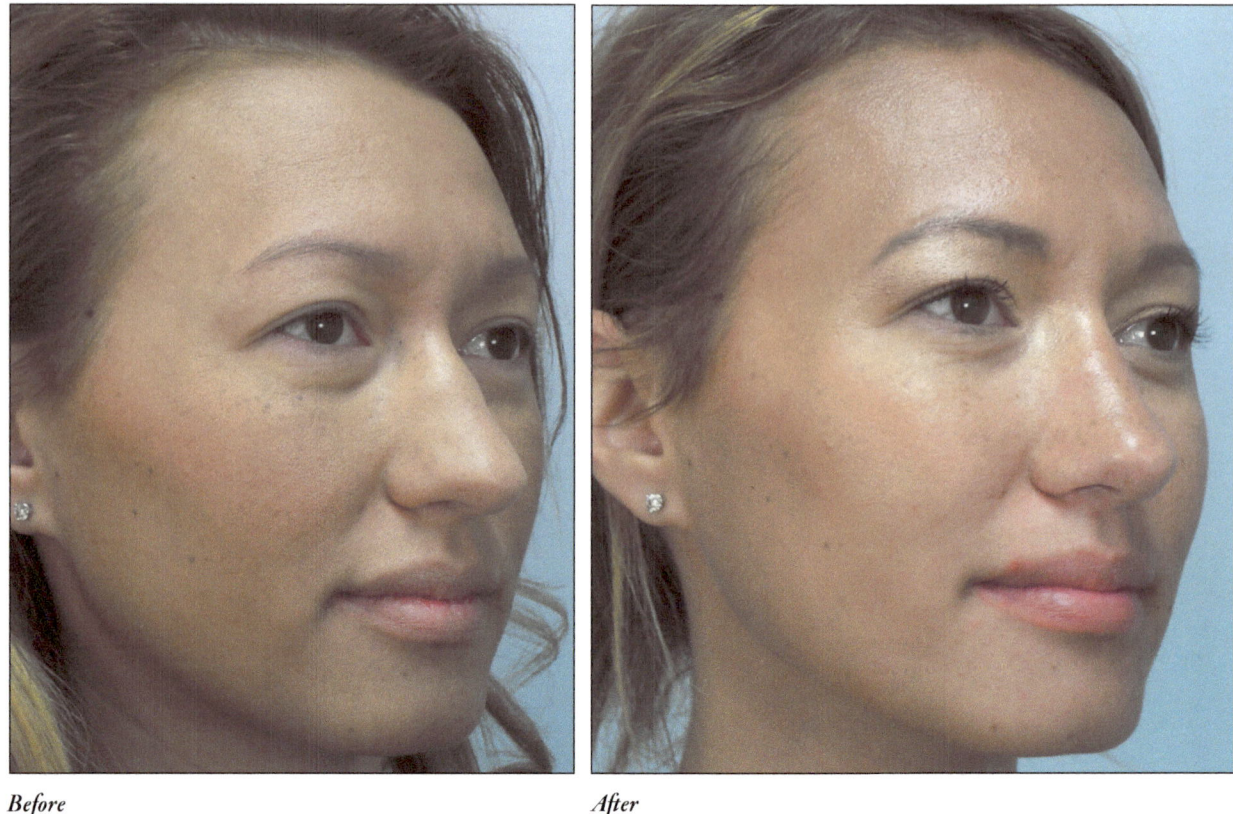

Before   *After*

THICK SKIN OF THE NOSE, WIDE, DROOPY, SLIGHTLY OVER PROJECTED NASAL TIP

The results reveal a less overprojected, droopy tip with a slightly opened nasolabial angle (angle of the nose/lip junction). The patient's nose has a more triangular appearance, creating a more aesthetically pleasing nose that fits her face and blends with her profile and with a strong framework intact (see following page).

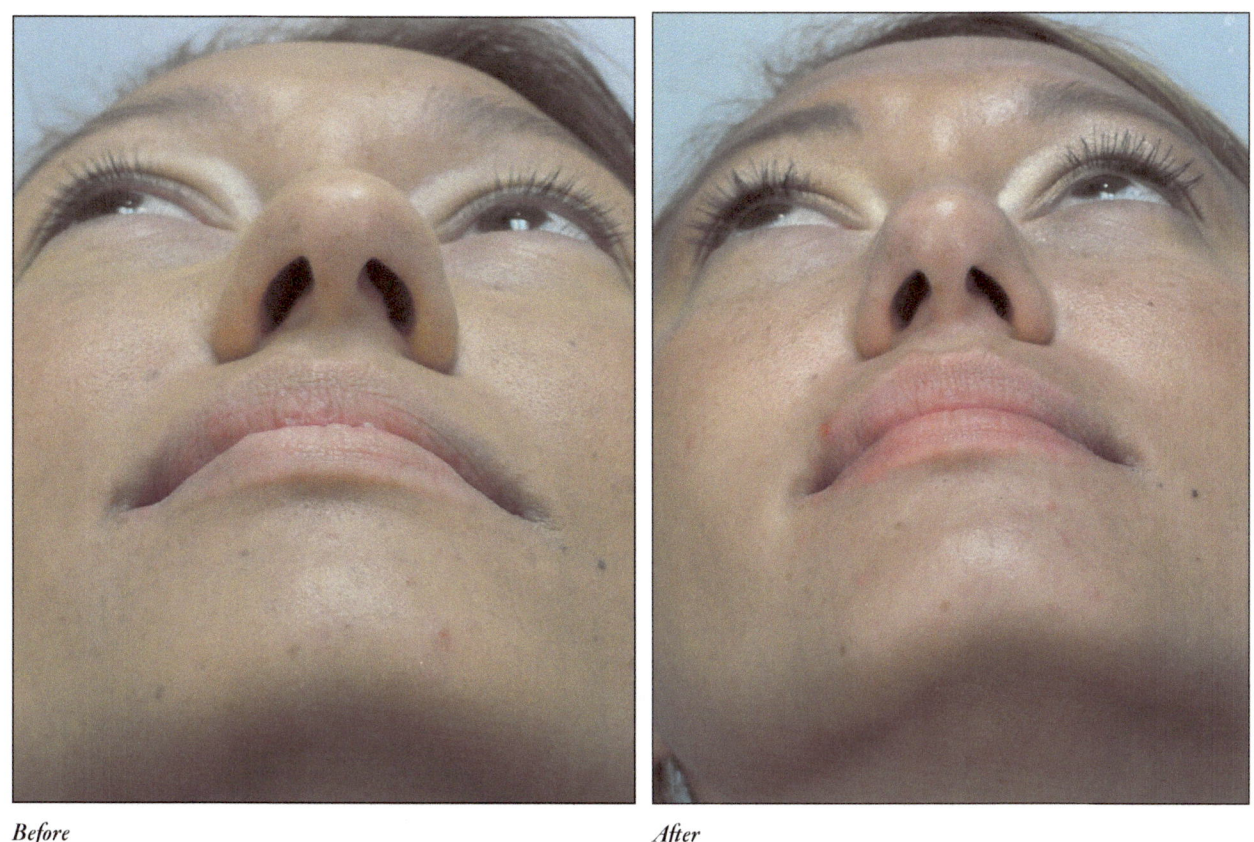

Before   *After*

THICK SKIN OF THE NOSE, WIDE, DROOPY, SLIGHTLY OVER PROJECTED NASAL TIP

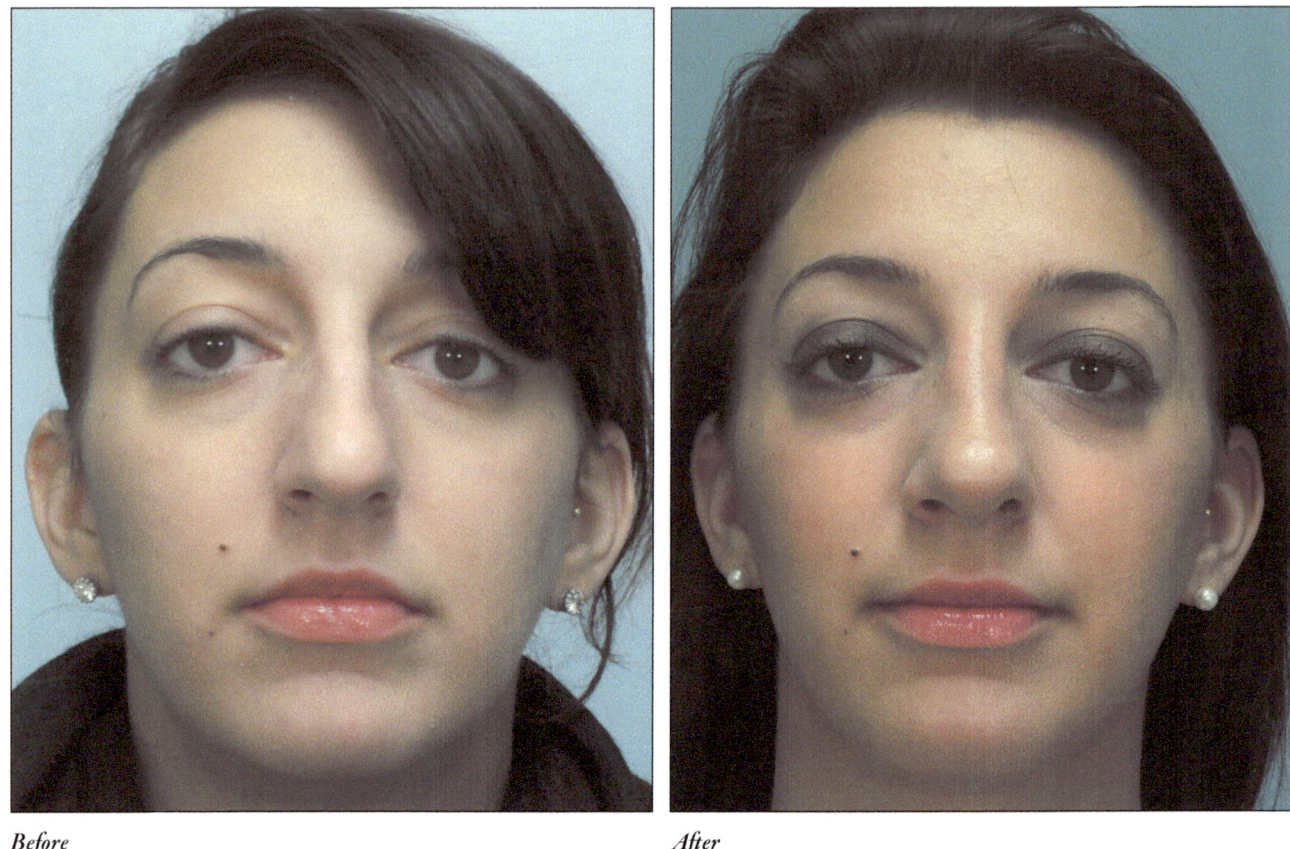

Before   *After*

DROOPY, OVER PROJECTED TIP WITH THICKER SKIN AND A NASAL BUMP

Patient's nose has a somewhat bulbous tip, which draws unwanted attention to it. This conservative improvement creates a very natural and aesthetically balanced face and draws attention to her entire face rather than her nose.

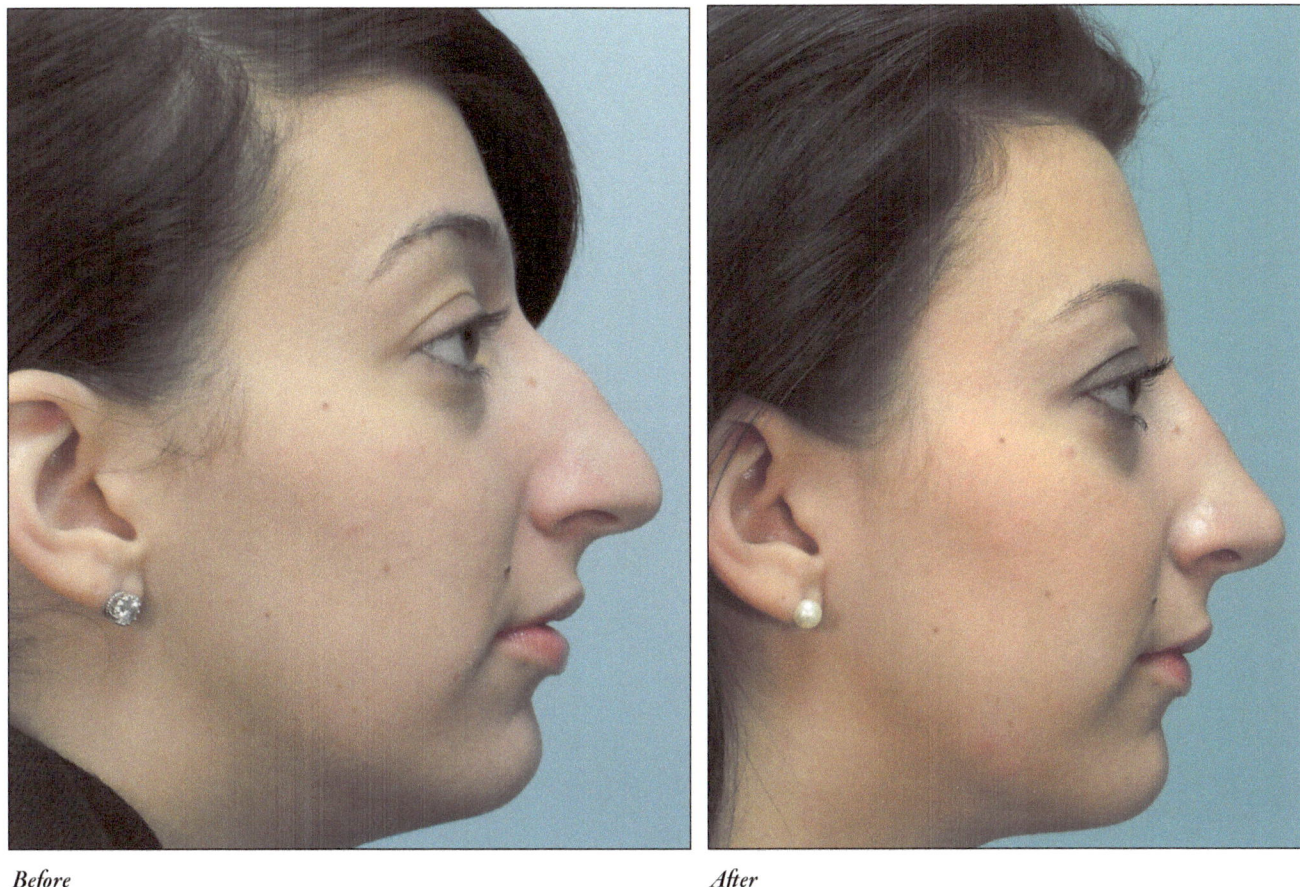

Before

After

DROOPY, OVER PROJECTED TIP WITH THICKER SKIN AND A NASAL BUMP

During rhinoplasty her nose tip was rotated slightly, reducing projection and better aligning her profile by reducing her nasal bump as seen here and on the following pages.

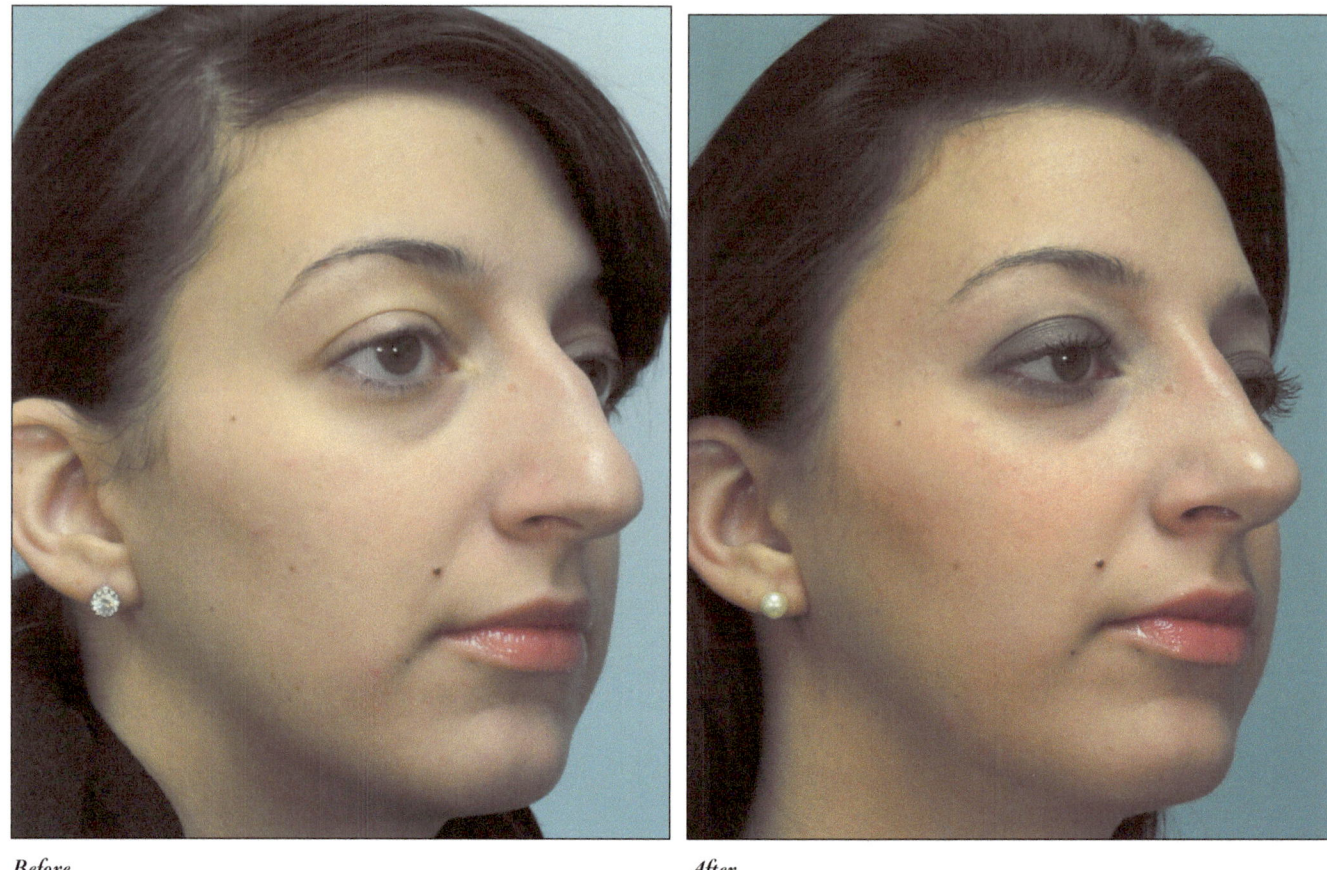

Before   *After*

DROOPY, OVER PROJECTED TIP WITH THICKER SKIN AND A NASAL BUMP

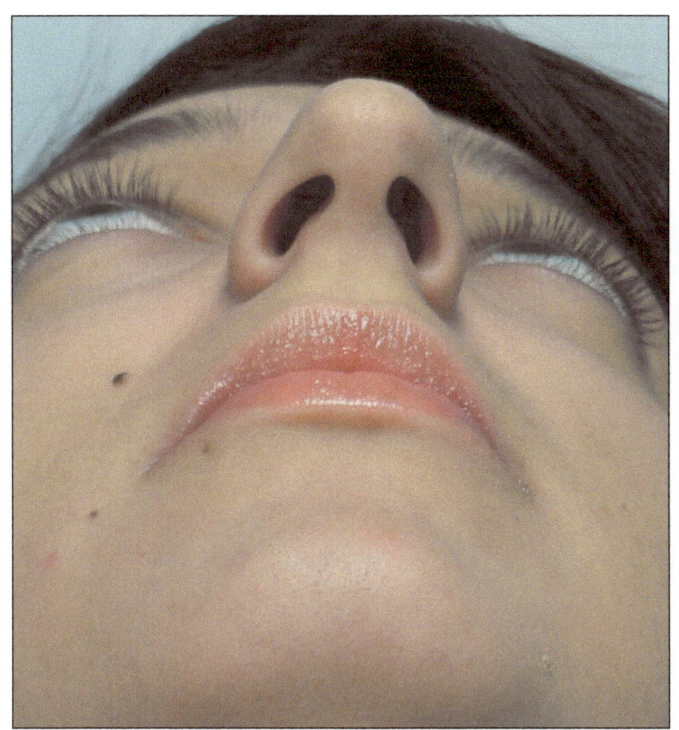
Before

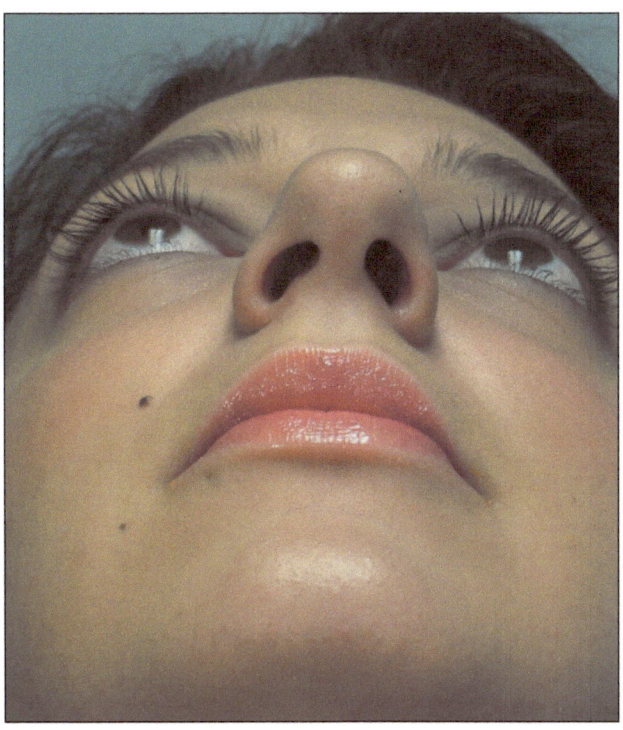
After

DROOPY, OVER PROJECTED TIP WITH THICKER SKIN AND A NASAL BUMP

 http://www.youtube.com/watch?v=Y1VKqSuoS8M&list=PL4CDA45694188ABB0&index=62

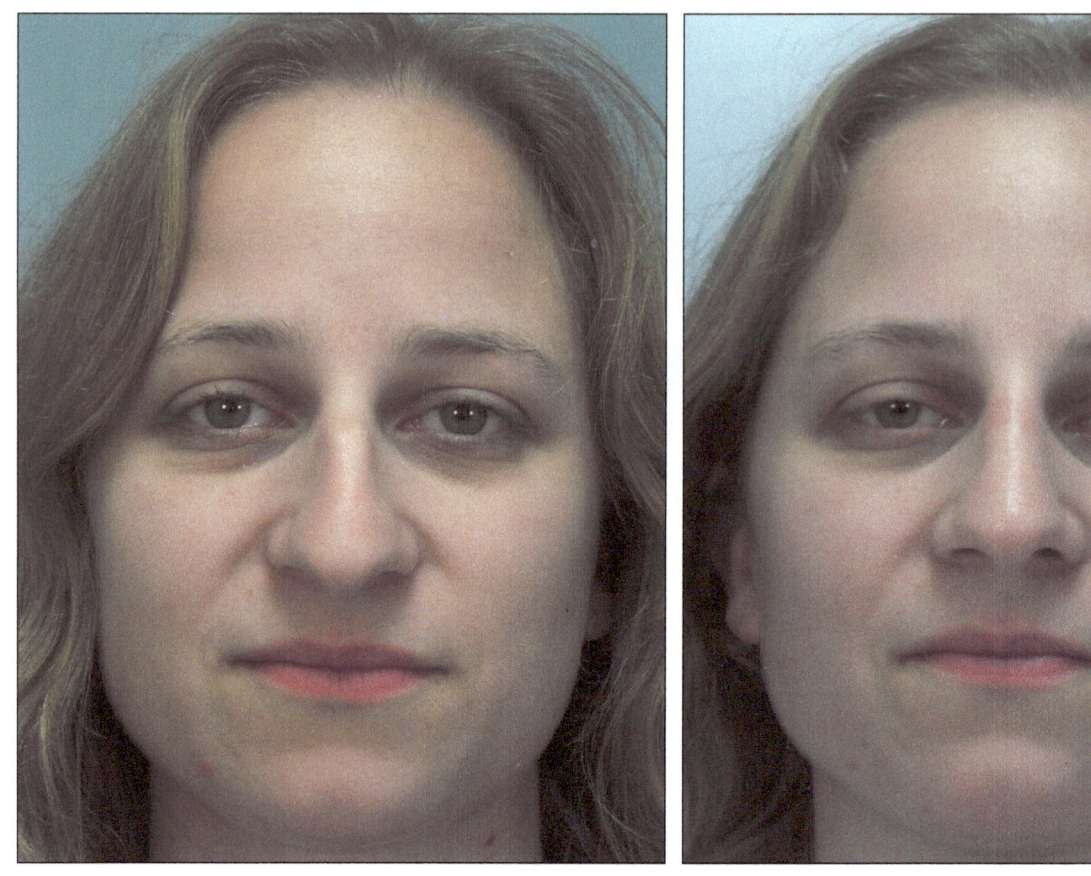

Before   *After*

LARGE, OVERPROJECTED TIP WITH HANGING COLUMELLA AND LARGE DORSAL BUMP

This patient had trouble breathing and was self-conscious about the appearance of her nose. Her front shows irregularities along the dorsum with a pinched middle vault (middle third of the nose). She also had a lack of tip definition, which created a more masculine nose.

This patient now has a more natural-looking nose that allows her to breathe more freely and better fits her face.

With rhinoplasty we created a much narrower nose tip while maintaining width from top to bottom and correcting the pinched look in the middle third.

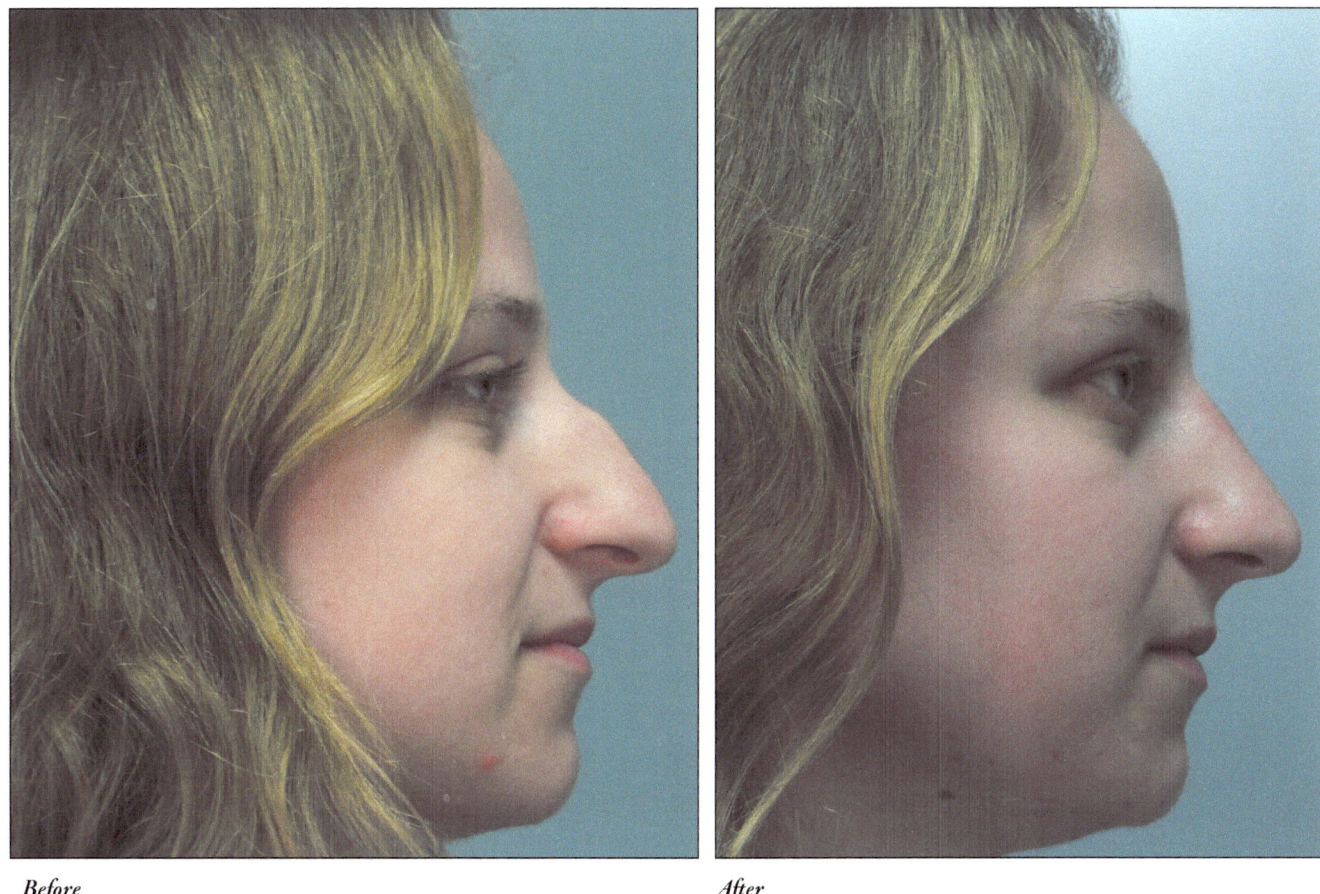

Before   *After*

LARGE, OVERPROJECTED TIP WITH HANGING COLUMELLA AND LARGE DORSAL BUMP

Her side view shows less of a droopy columella (nostril region) and nasal bump. The tip of the nose has been rotated up approximately ten degrees as seen here and on the following pages.

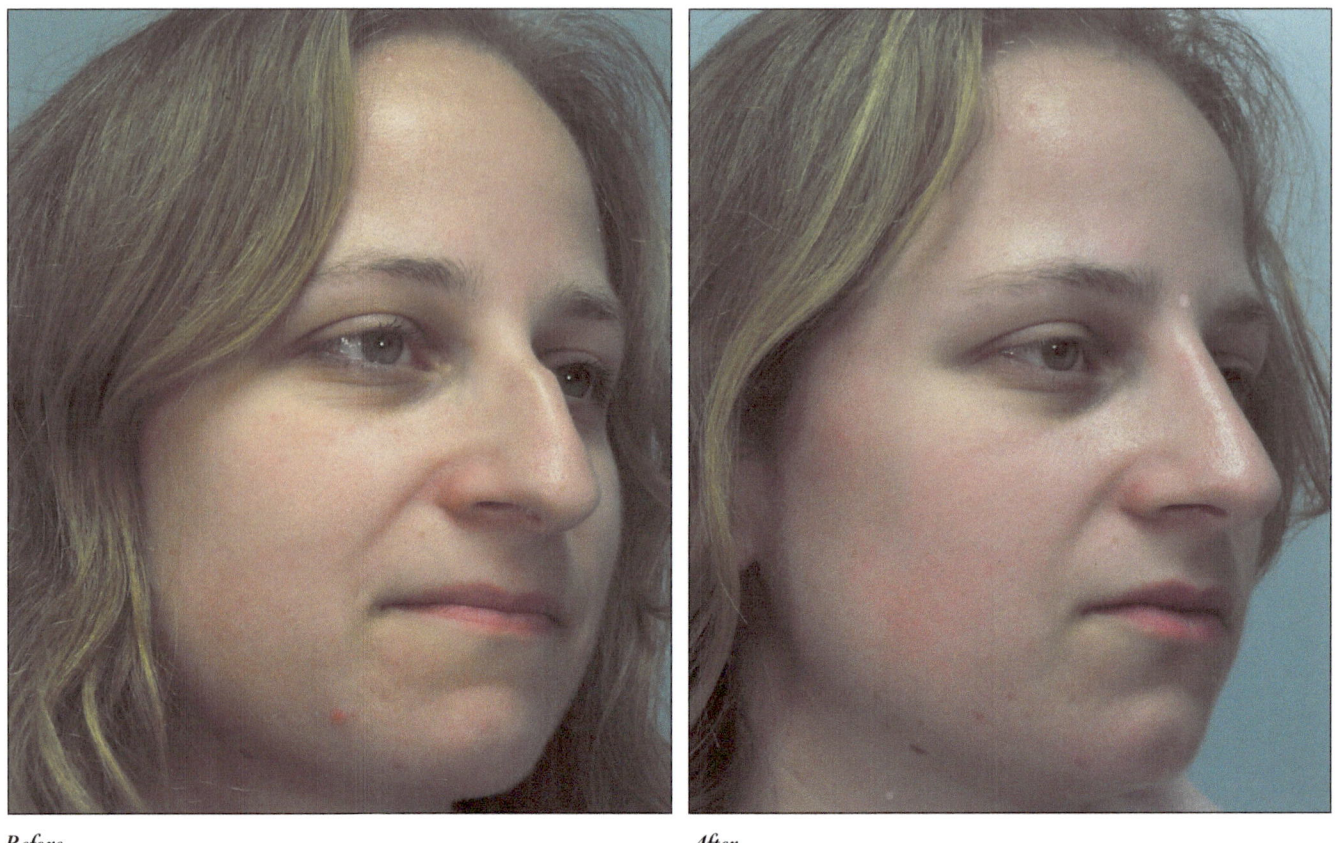

Before   *After*

LARGE, OVERPROJECTED TIP WITH HANGING COLUMELLA AND LARGE DORSAL BUMP

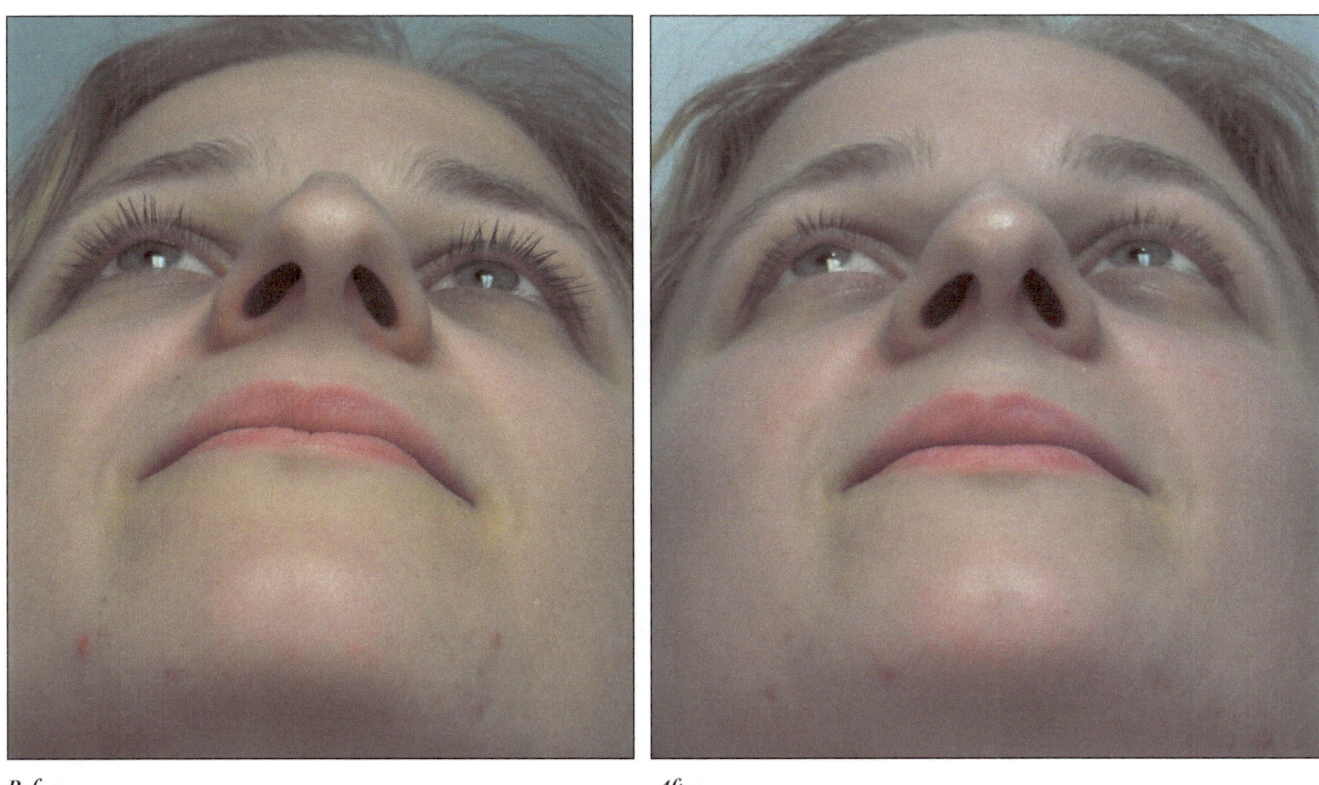

Before   *After*

LARGE, OVERPROJECTED TIP WITH HANGING COLUMELLA AND LARGE DORSAL BUMP

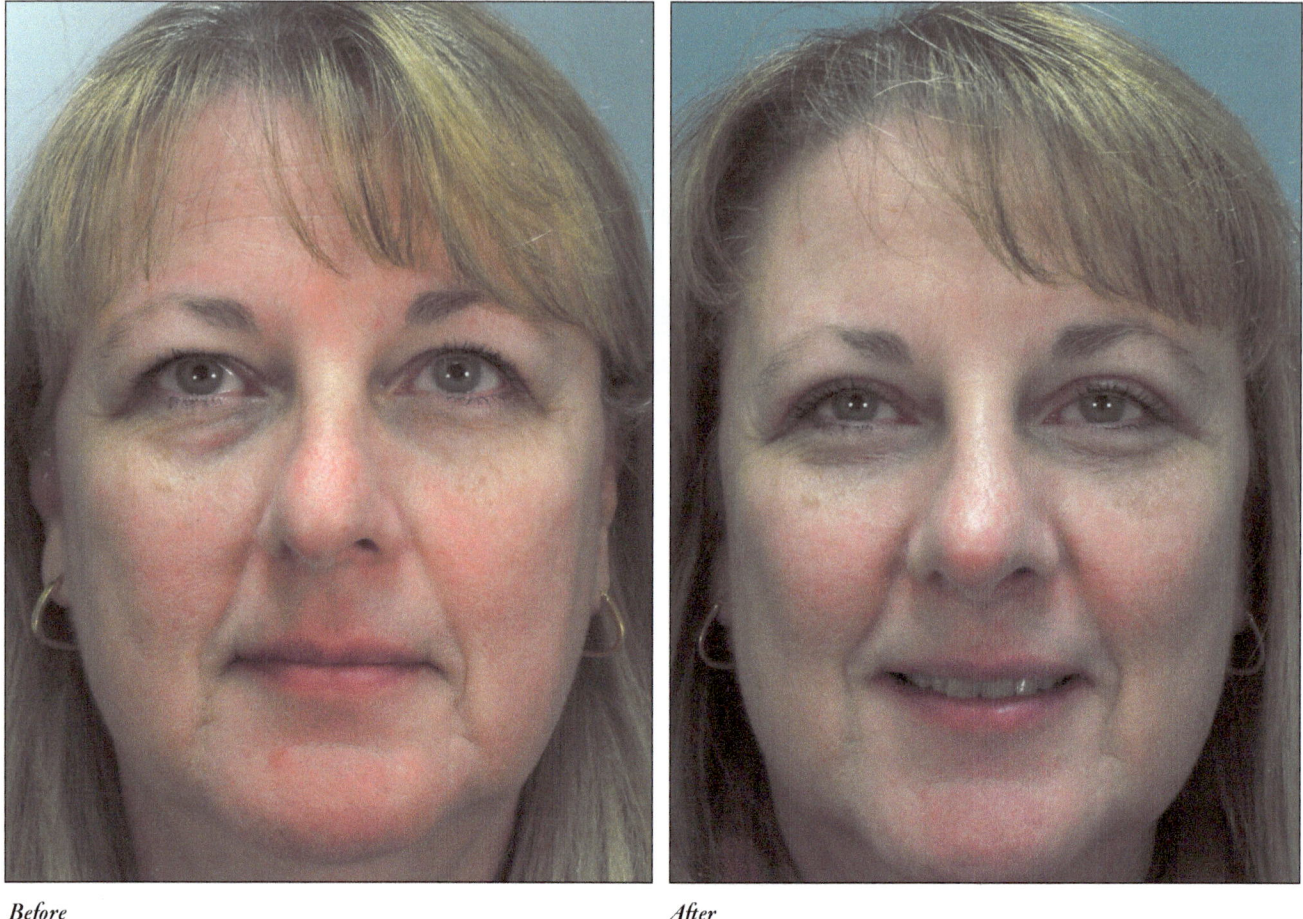

Before   *After*

THICKER SKIN AND DROOPY TIP, CROOKED NOSE

This is a mature patient that has a crooked nose and thick skin, which limits the definition that can be achieved in rhinoplasty.

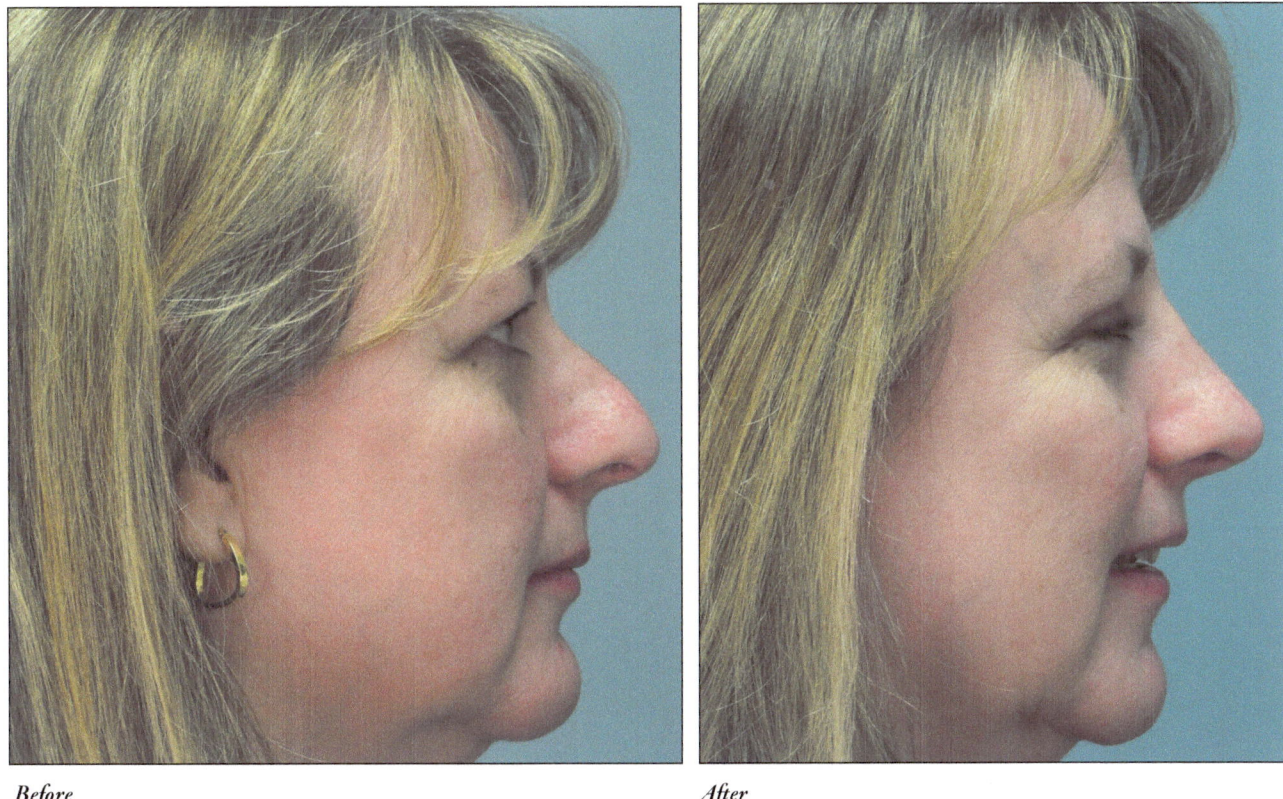

Before　　　　　　　　　　　　　　　　　　　　*After*

THICKER SKIN AND DROOPY TIP, CROOKED NOSE

However by rotating and correcting the patient's droopy tip, the result is a more aesthetically pleasing profile. This results in a less projected tip that fits her face while creating a more youthful appearance.

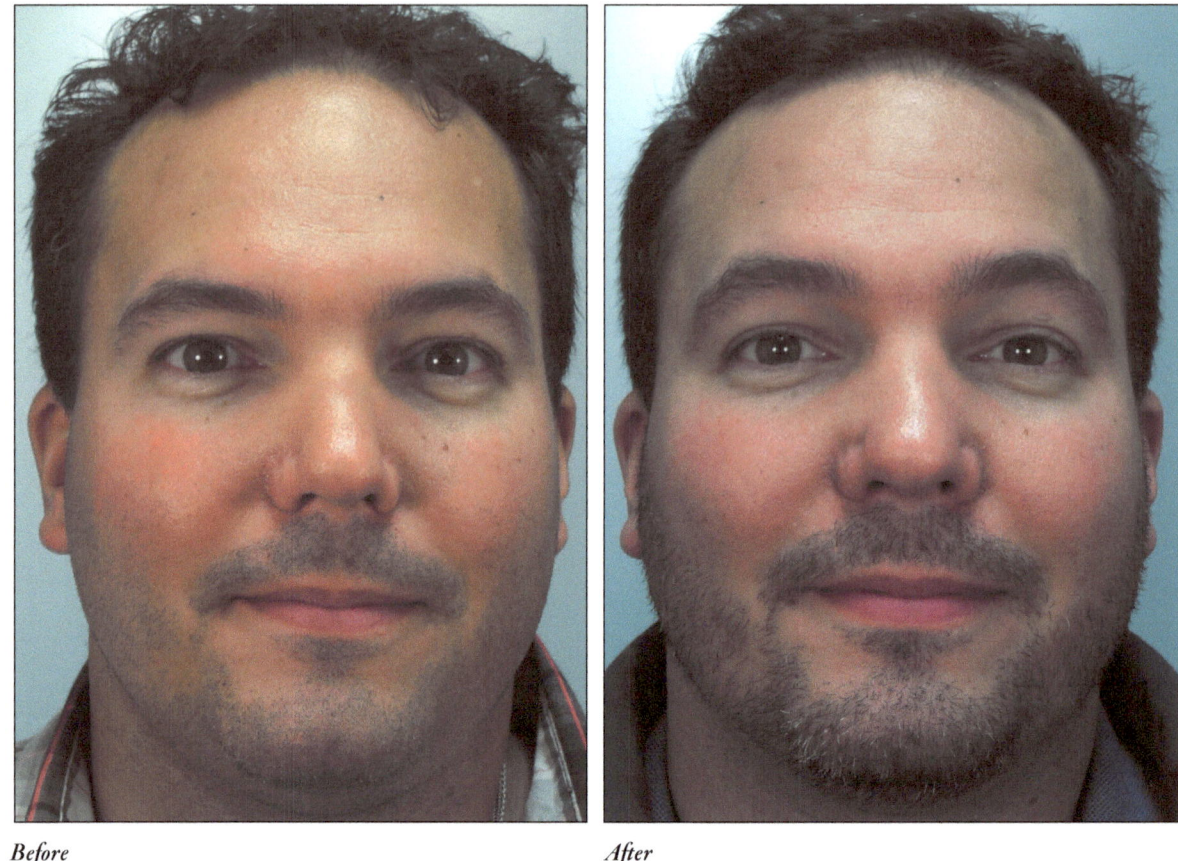

Before   *After*

REVISION RHINOPLASTY WITH COSTAL (RIB) CARTILAGE

This patient had previous nasal surgery which left him with a "boxer's nose" that did not function well.

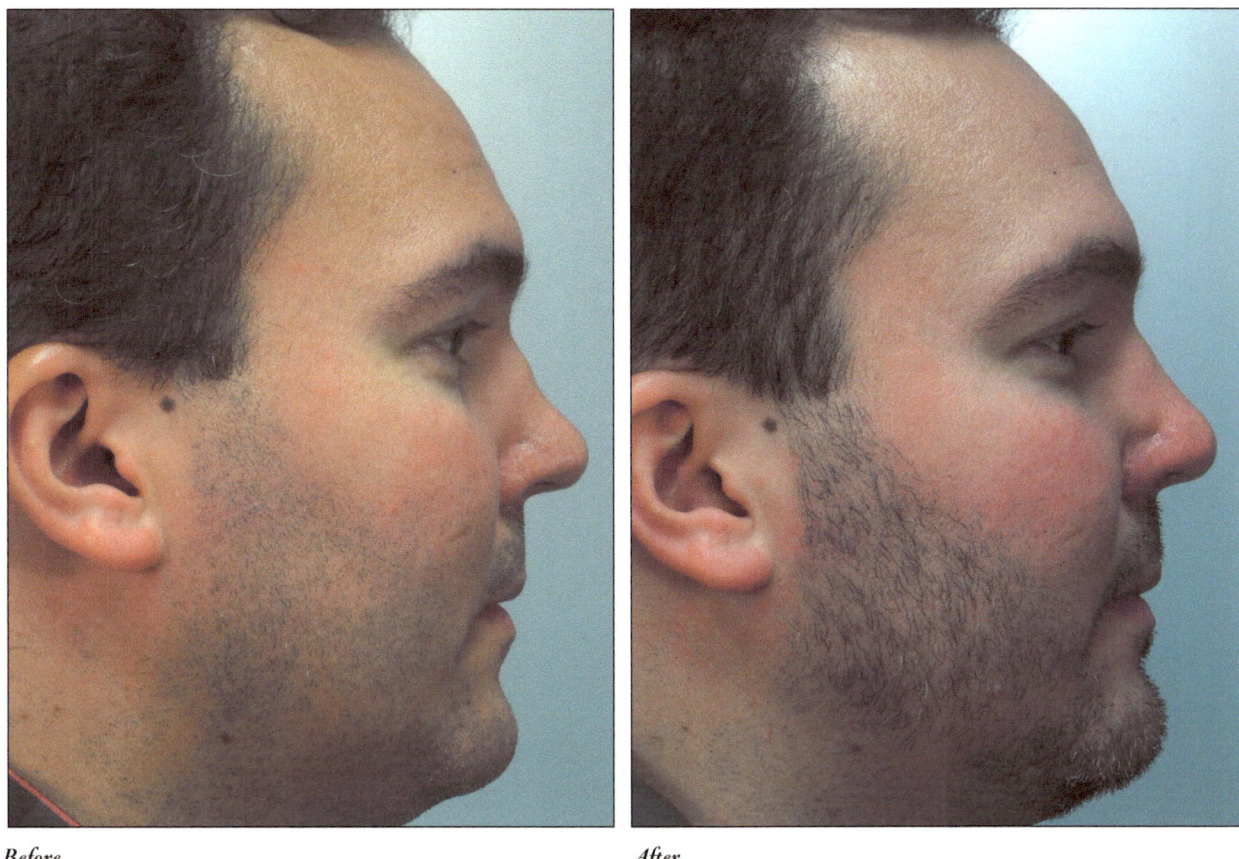

Before   *After*

REVISION RHINOPLASTY WITH COSTAL (RIB) CARTILAGE

Since the patient had no additional useful cartilage in the septum of the nose, he decided to proceed with revision rhinoplasty using a small amount of rib cartilage from the breast. The cartilage is fashioned and carved to rebuild the nose as shown here and on the following pages.

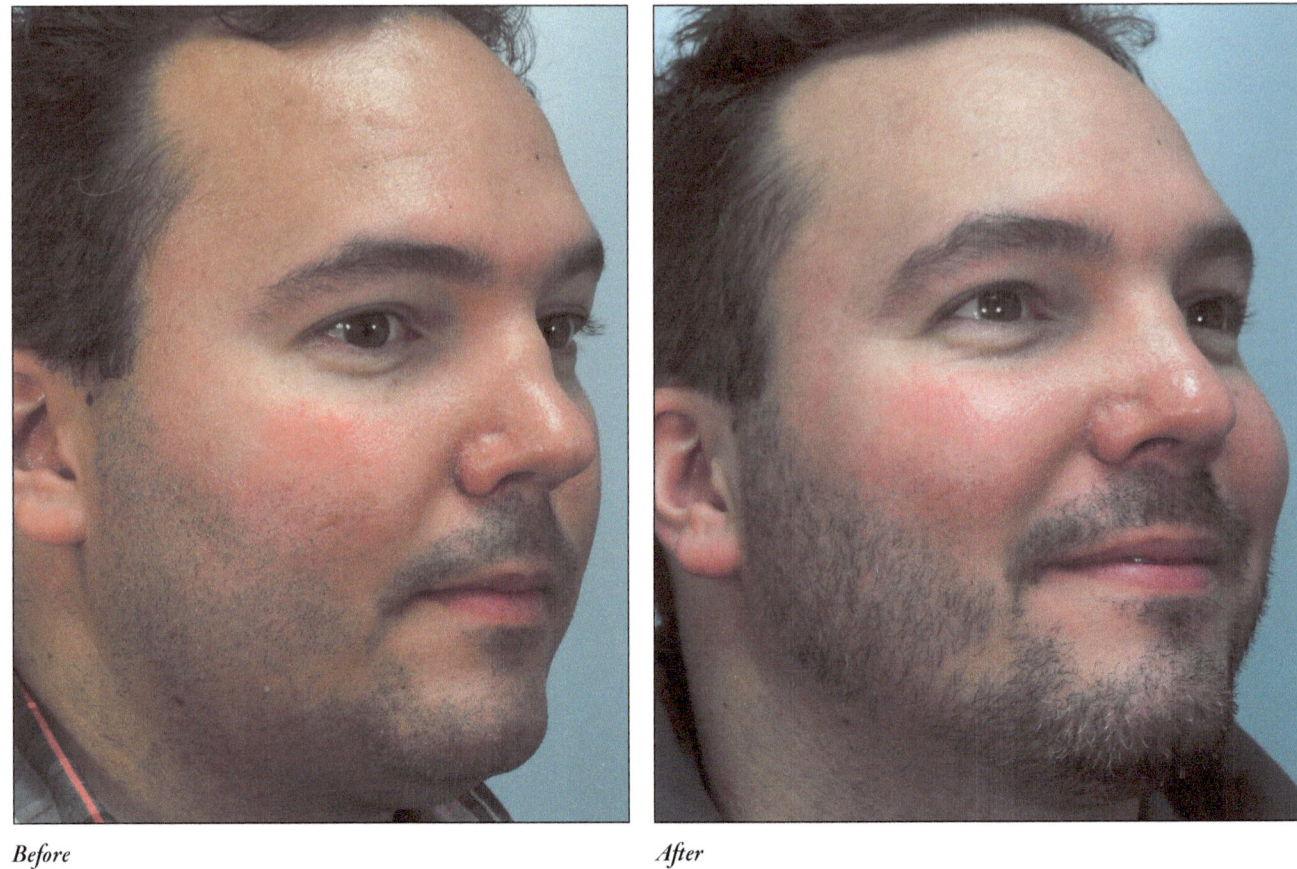

Before

After

REVISION RHINOPLASTY WITH COSTAL (RIB) CARTILAGE

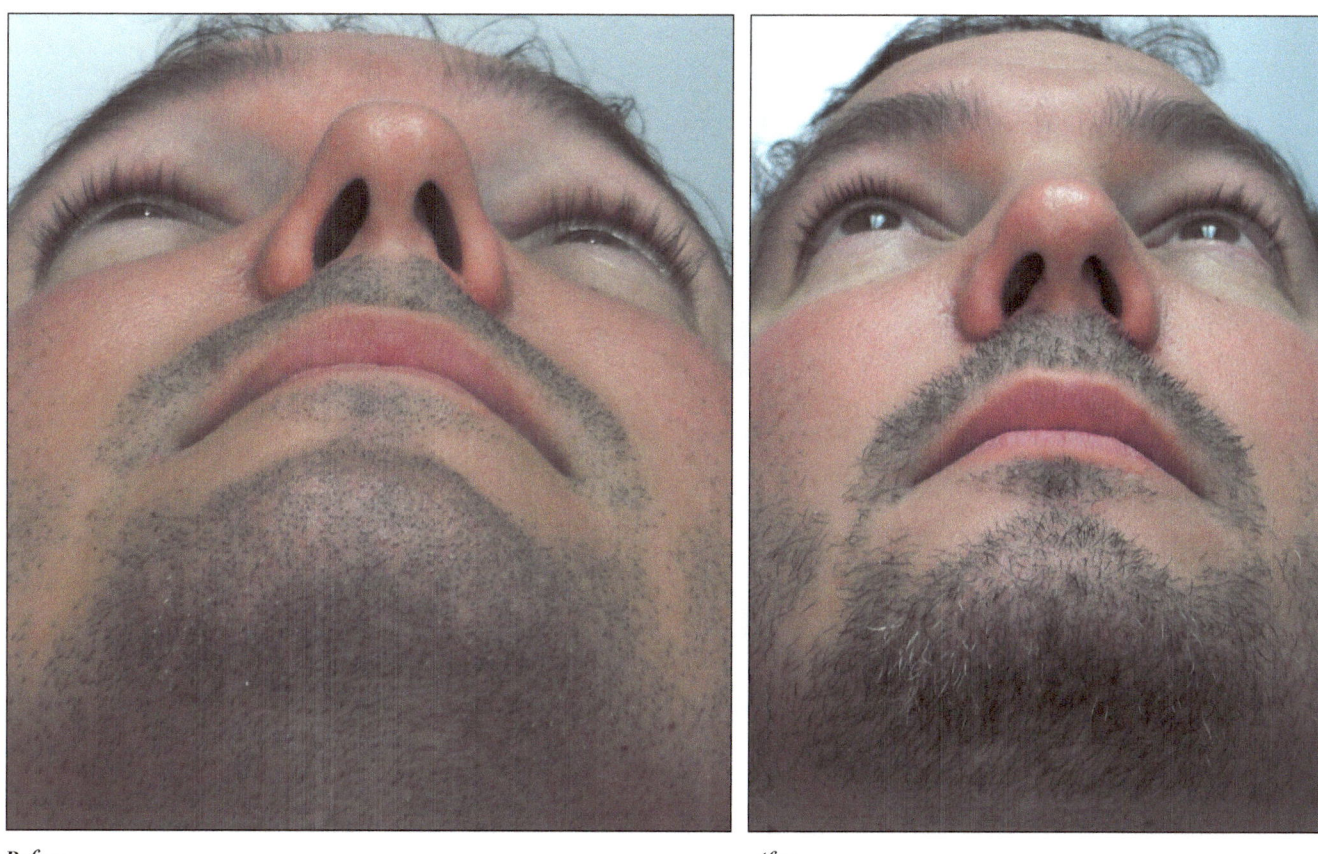

Before   *After*

REVISION RHINOPLASTY WITH COSTAL (RIB) CARTILAGE

The procedures were performed as an outpatient and resulted in a more natural-looking nose that fits his face with no evidence of previous trauma. This patient also experienced much improvement in his breathing.

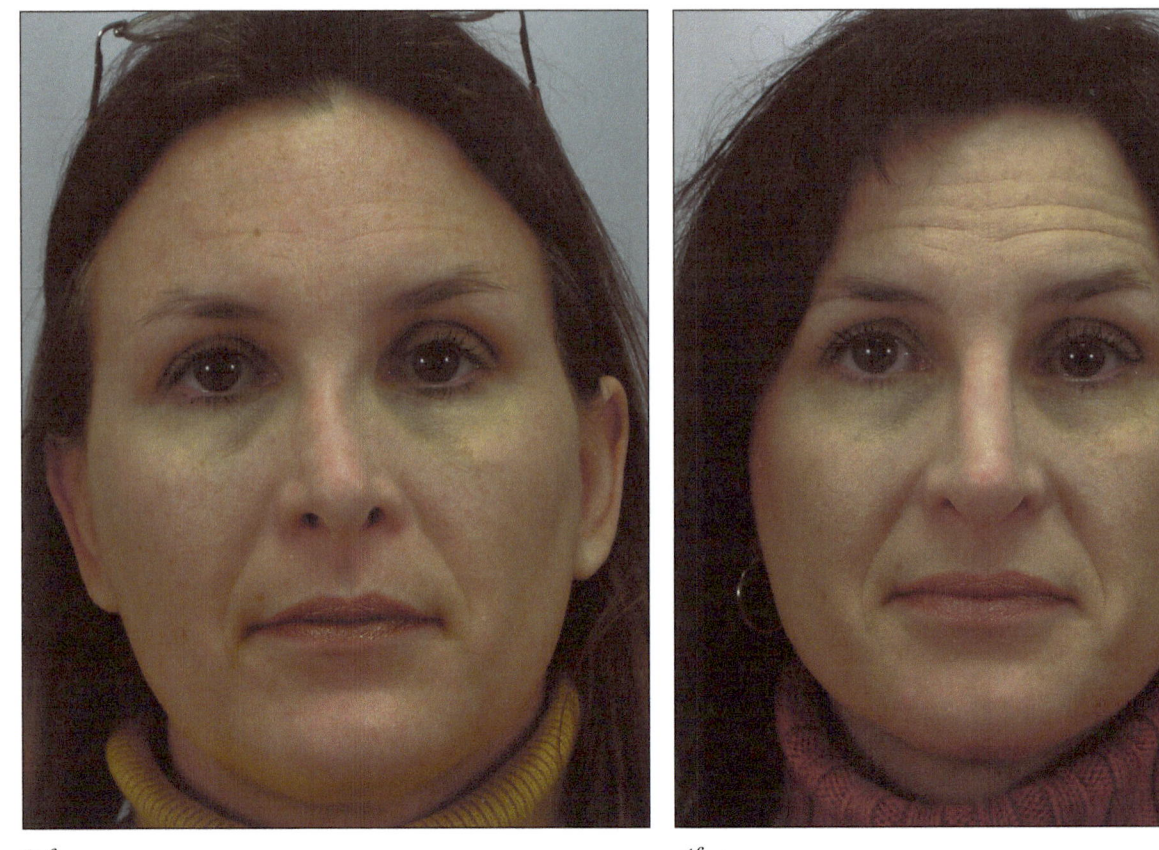

Before   *After*

SADDLE NOSE DEFORMITY AS A RESULT OF DOMESTIC VIOLENCE INJURY

This patient had previous surgery due to a physical injury associated with domestic violence. As you can see from her postoperative photos, her nose is much straighter with a more normal appearance.

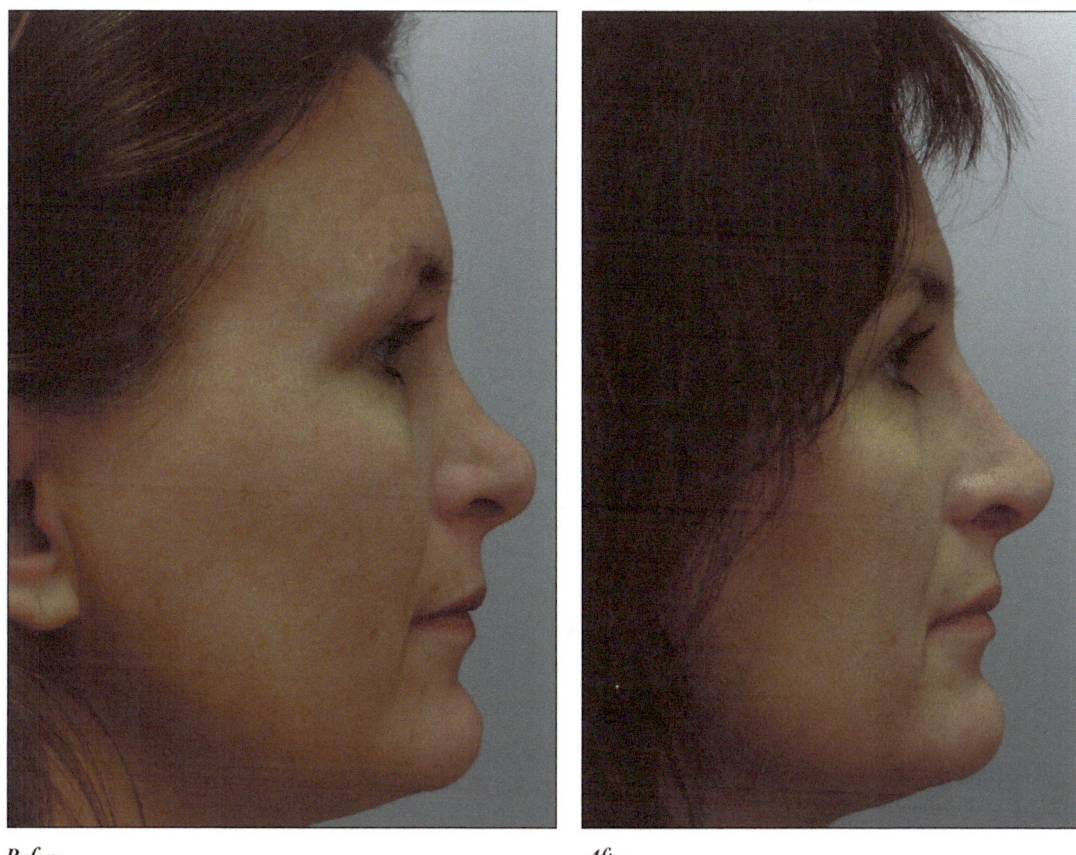

Before   *After*

SADDLE NOSE DEFORMITY AS A RESULT OF DOMESTIC VIOLENCE INJURY

This patient underwent a cosmetic revision rhinoplasty, using cartilage harvested from her ears, to rebuild her profile, nasal base (as seen here and on the following pages) and, as important in such cases, her self-esteem.

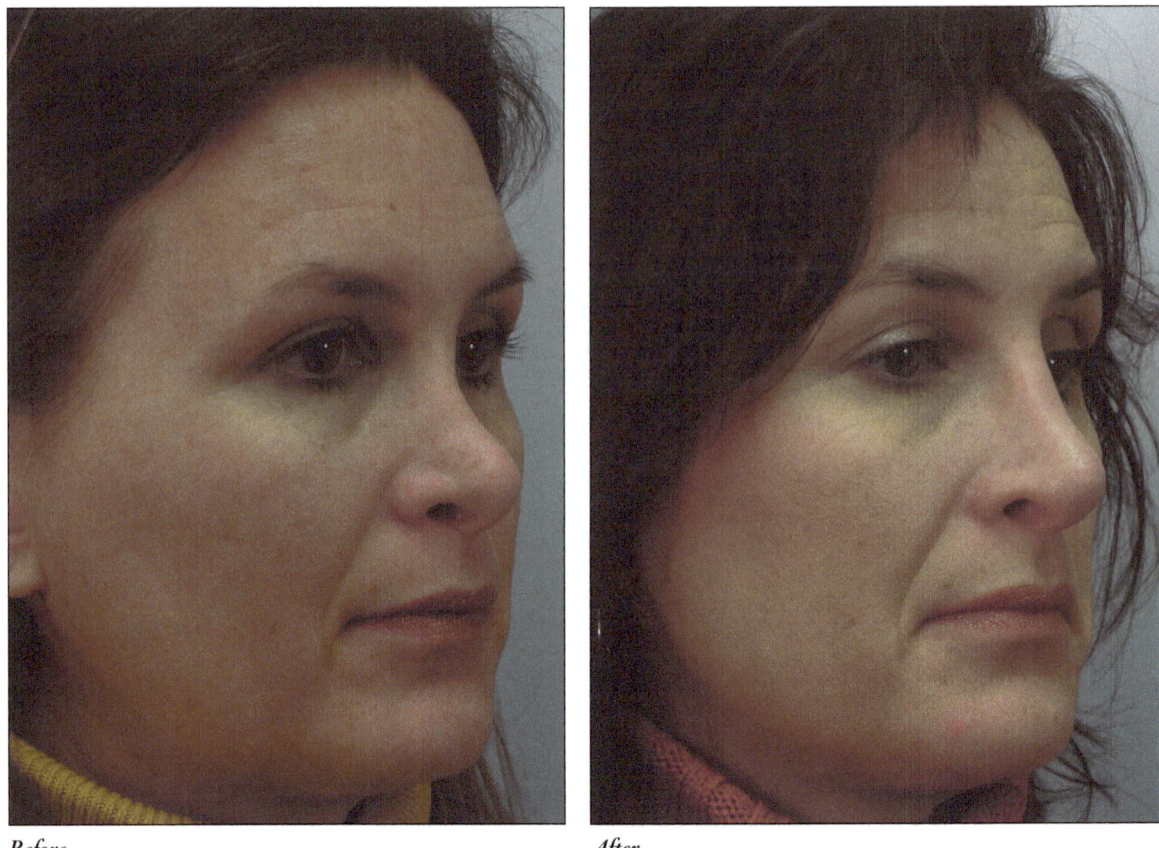

Before

After

SADDLE NOSE DEFORMITY AS A RESULT OF DOMESTIC VIOLENCE INJURY

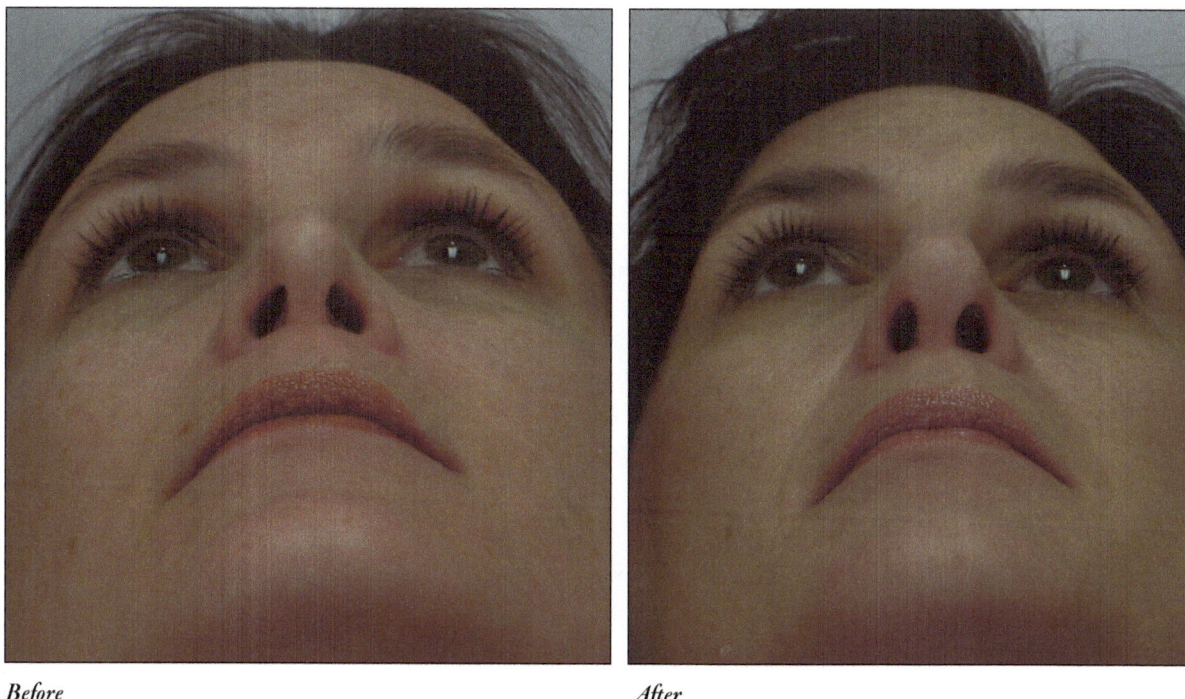

Before   *After*

SADDLE NOSE DEFORMITY AS A RESULT OF DOMESTIC VIOLENCE INJURY

This patient benefited from the American Academy of Facial Plastic and Reconstructive Surgery (AAFPRS) Domestic Violence Program, offered through my practice and others. Today, years after her surgery, she enjoys a much better life advocating and acting as a spokesperson for the program.

 http://www.youtube.com/watch?v=v34PAIkJVMA&list=PL4CDA45694188ABB0&index=26

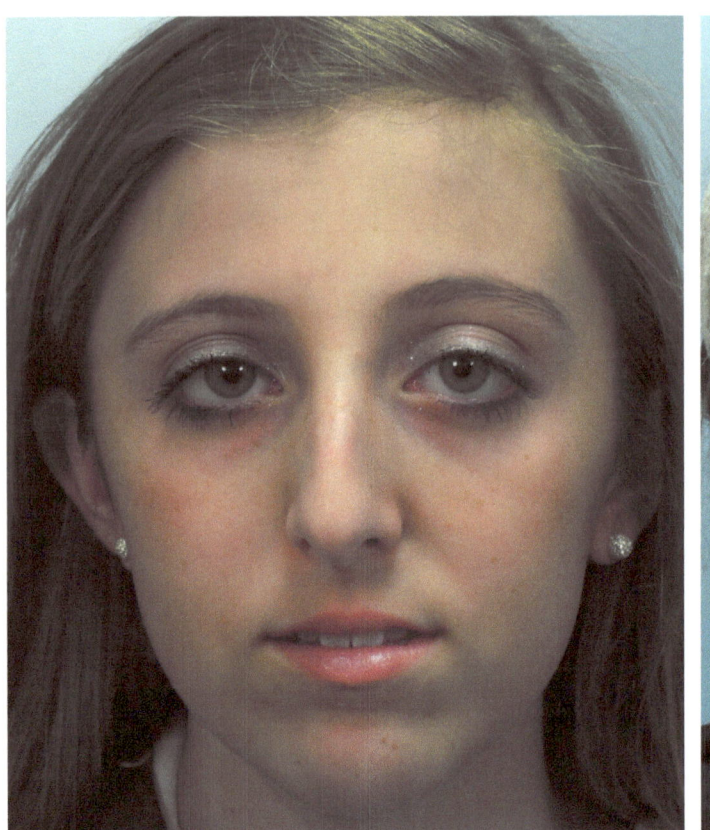
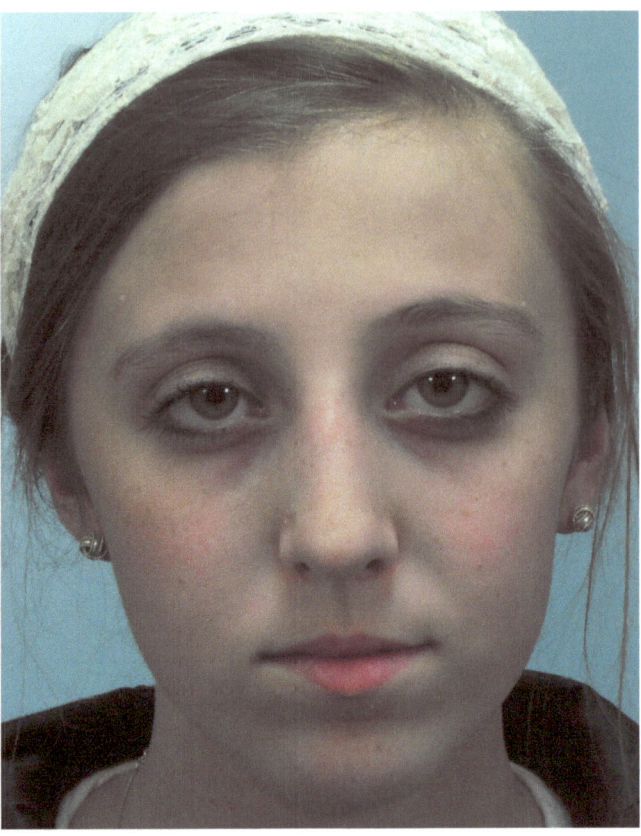

Before　　　　　　　　　　　　　　　　　　　　　*After*

CROOKED NOSE, NARROW MIDDLE VAULT, OVERPROJECTED TIP, HANGING COLUMELLA, AND DORSAL BUMP

This teenager's nose was not only crooked but had a narrow middle vault, making it difficult to breathe.

With rhinoplasty we straightened her nose while widening the middle vault and narrowing the tip, giving her a nose that balances from top to bottom. The overall result is a more visually appealing nose, more in alignment with this young woman's face.

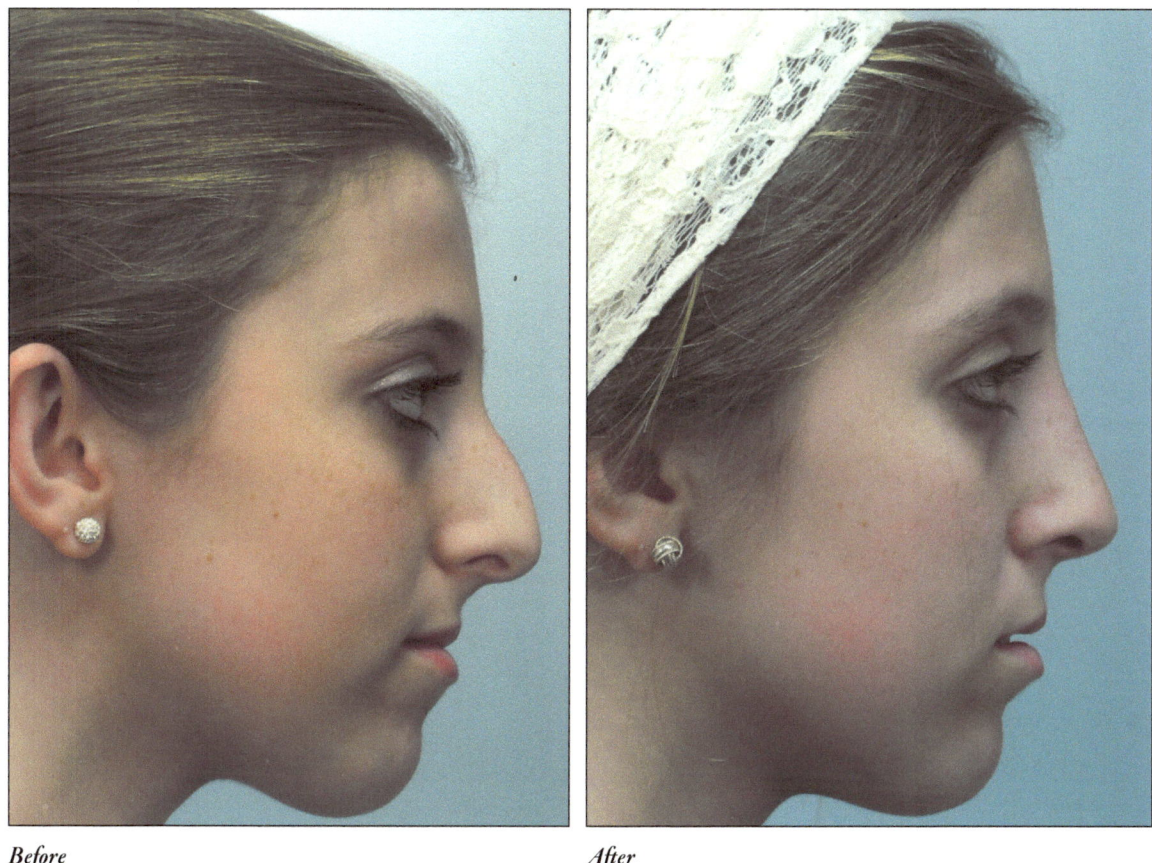

Before   *After*

CROOKED NOSE, NARROW MIDDLE VAULT, OVERPROJECTED TIP, HANGING COLUMELLA, AND DORSAL BUMP

The patient also had a bump and a droopy columella (middle nostril region) that took away from the appearance of her nose and created an illusion of a large nostril, causing her nose to further stand out from her other features.

The columella or nostril region has been tucked up, the nose tip rotated slightly, and the dorsal bump addressed as seen here and on the following pages.

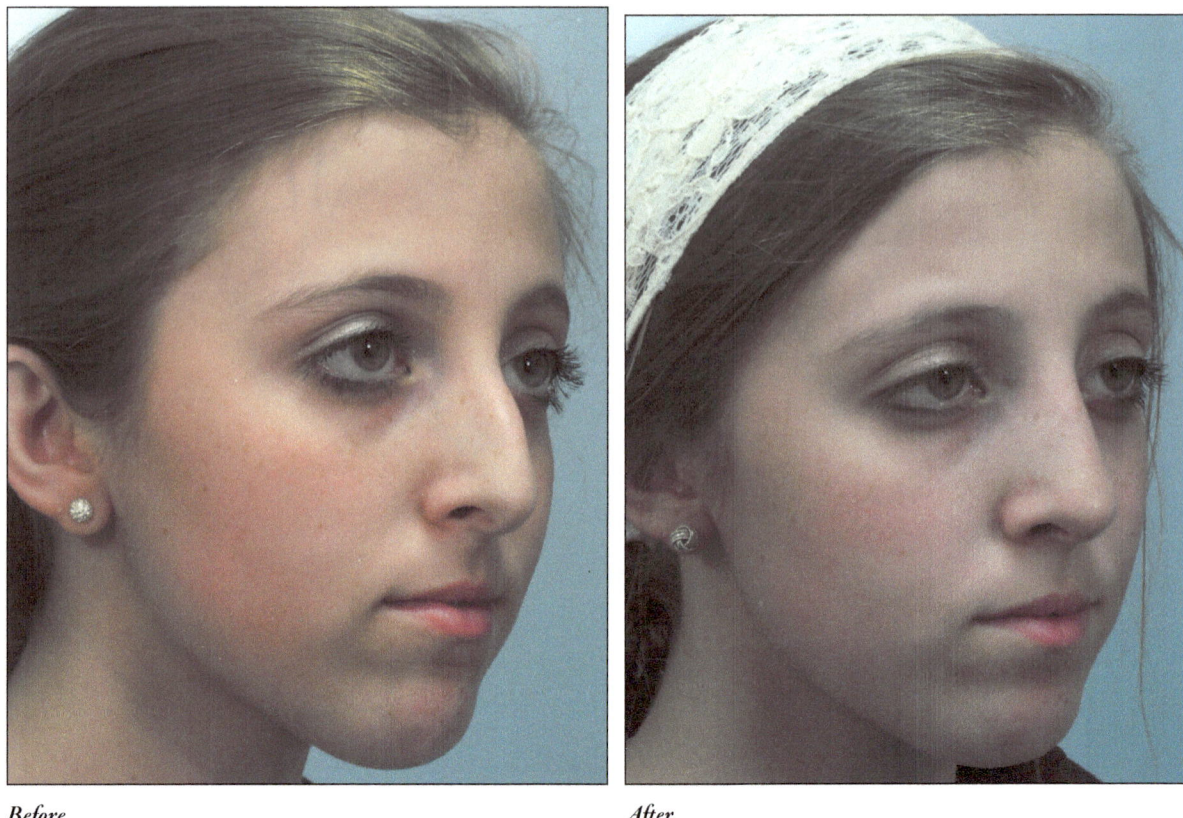

Before *After*

CROOKED NOSE, NARROW MIDDLE VAULT, OVERPROJECTED TIP, HANGING COLUMELLA, AND DORSAL BUMP

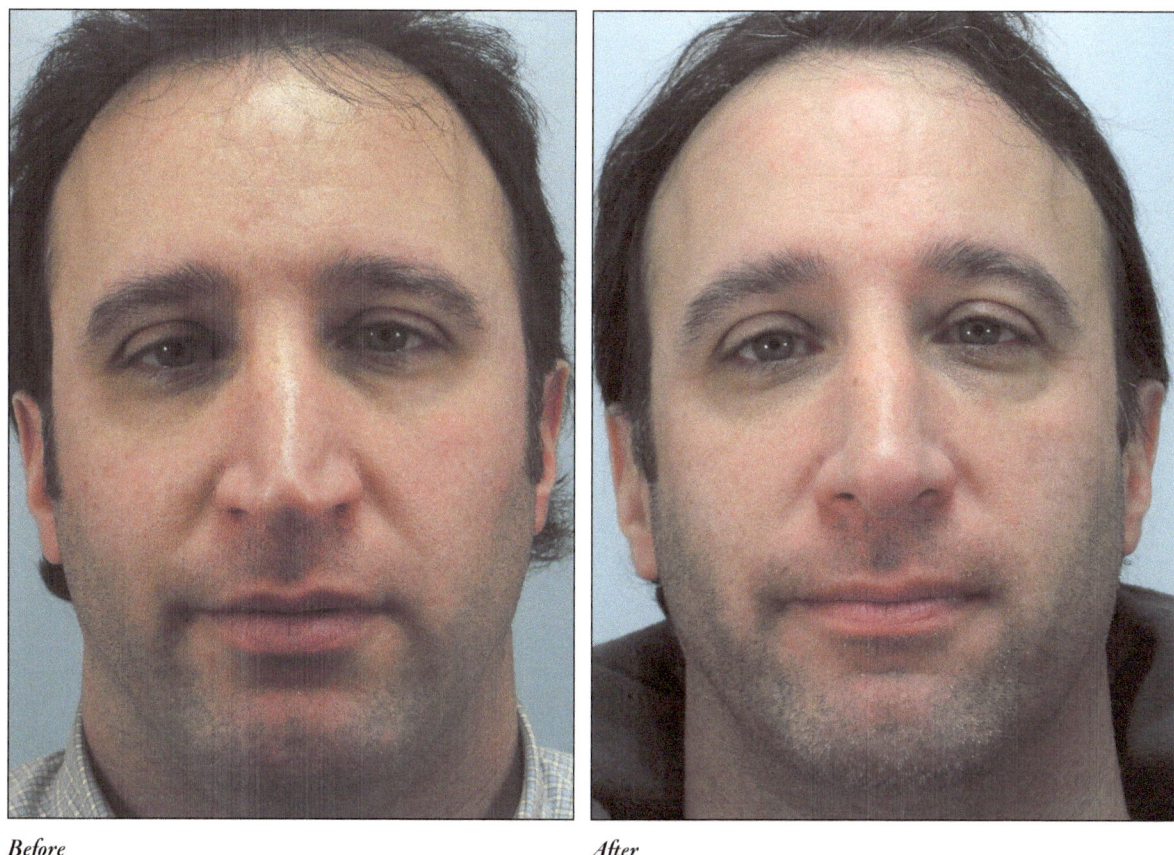

Before   *After*

PINCHED NASAL TIP, CROOKED DROOPY NOSE WITH A SLIGHT BUMP

Using an open approach rhinoplasty, this patient's nose is now much straighter, less droopy, and the tip is more in balance with the middle aspect and upper aspect of his nose as seen here and on the following pages.

This patient had been bothered by the pinched appearance of his nose, which also caused difficulty in breathing. He also now breathes easier.

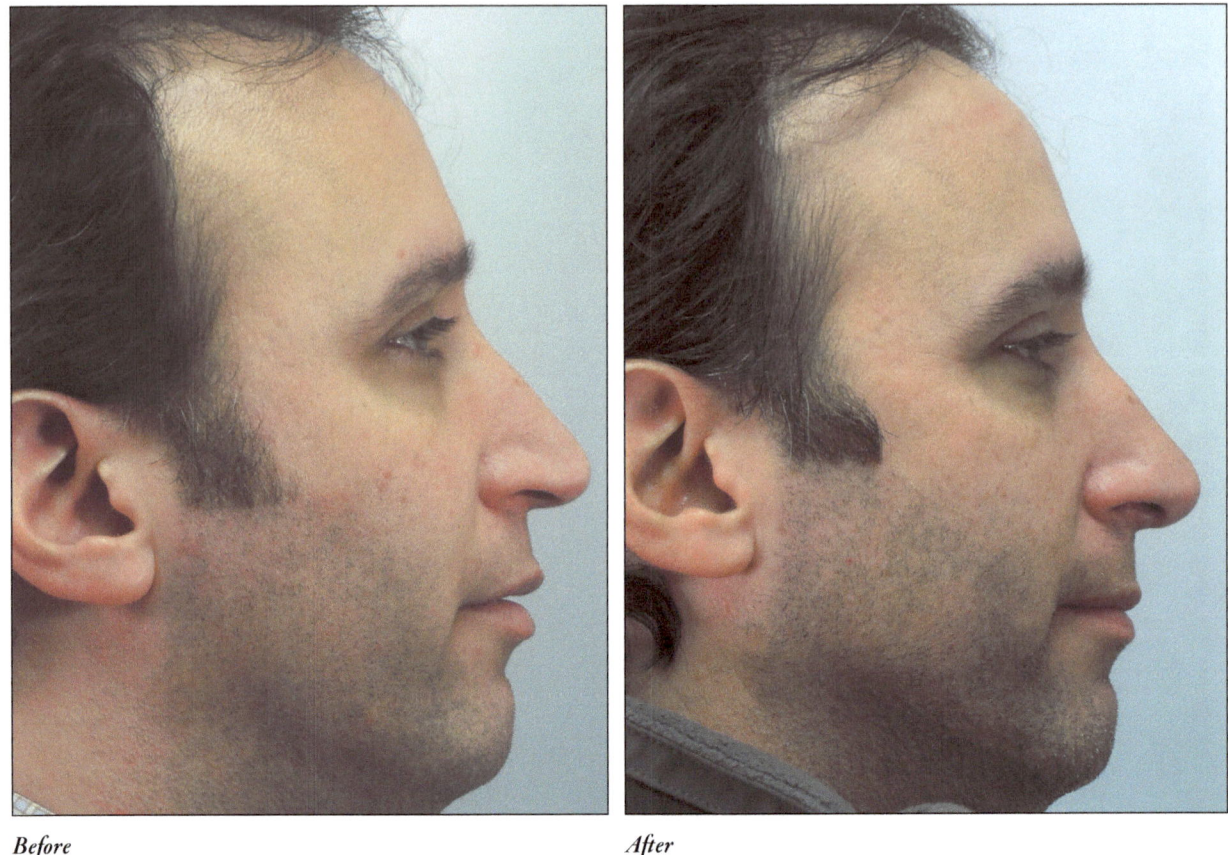

Before   *After*

PINCHED NASAL TIP, CROOKED DROOPY NOSE WITH A SLIGHT BUMP

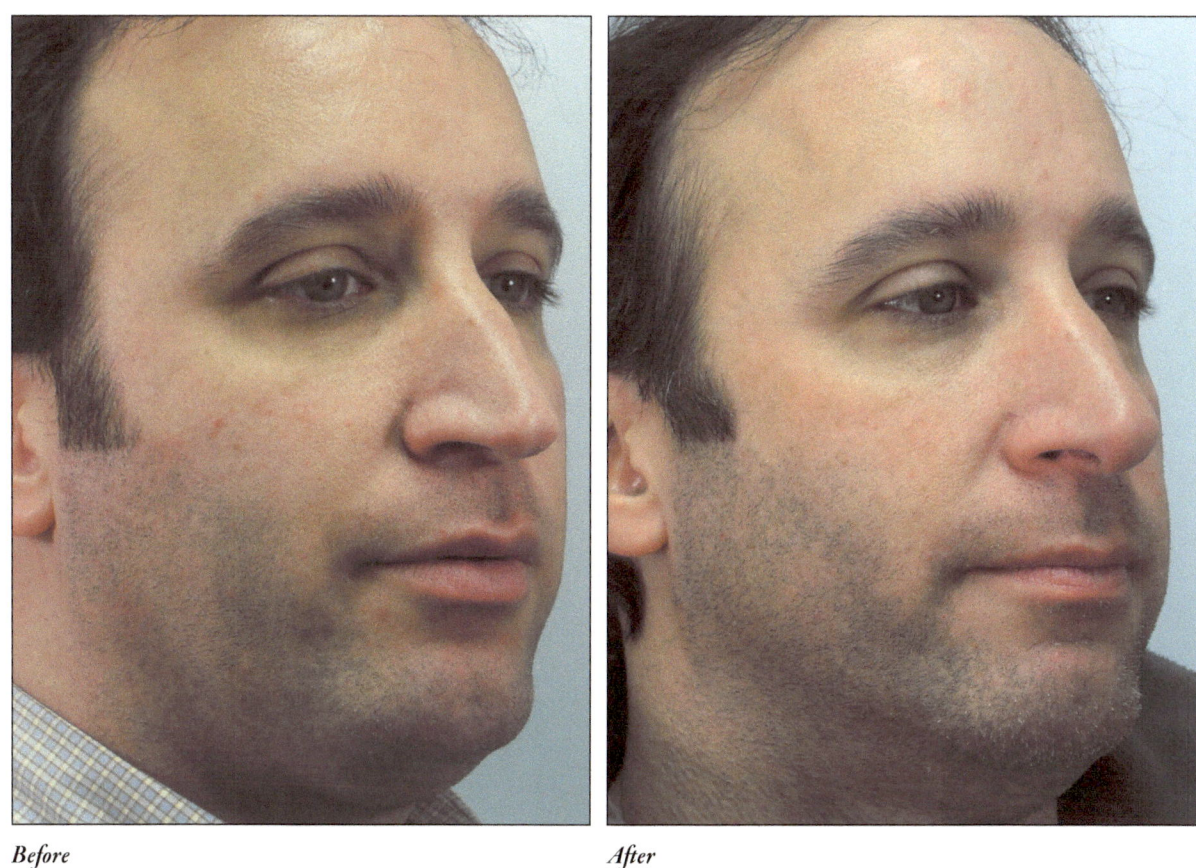

Before
After

PINCHED NASAL TIP, CROOKED DROOPY NOSE WITH A SLIGHT BUMP

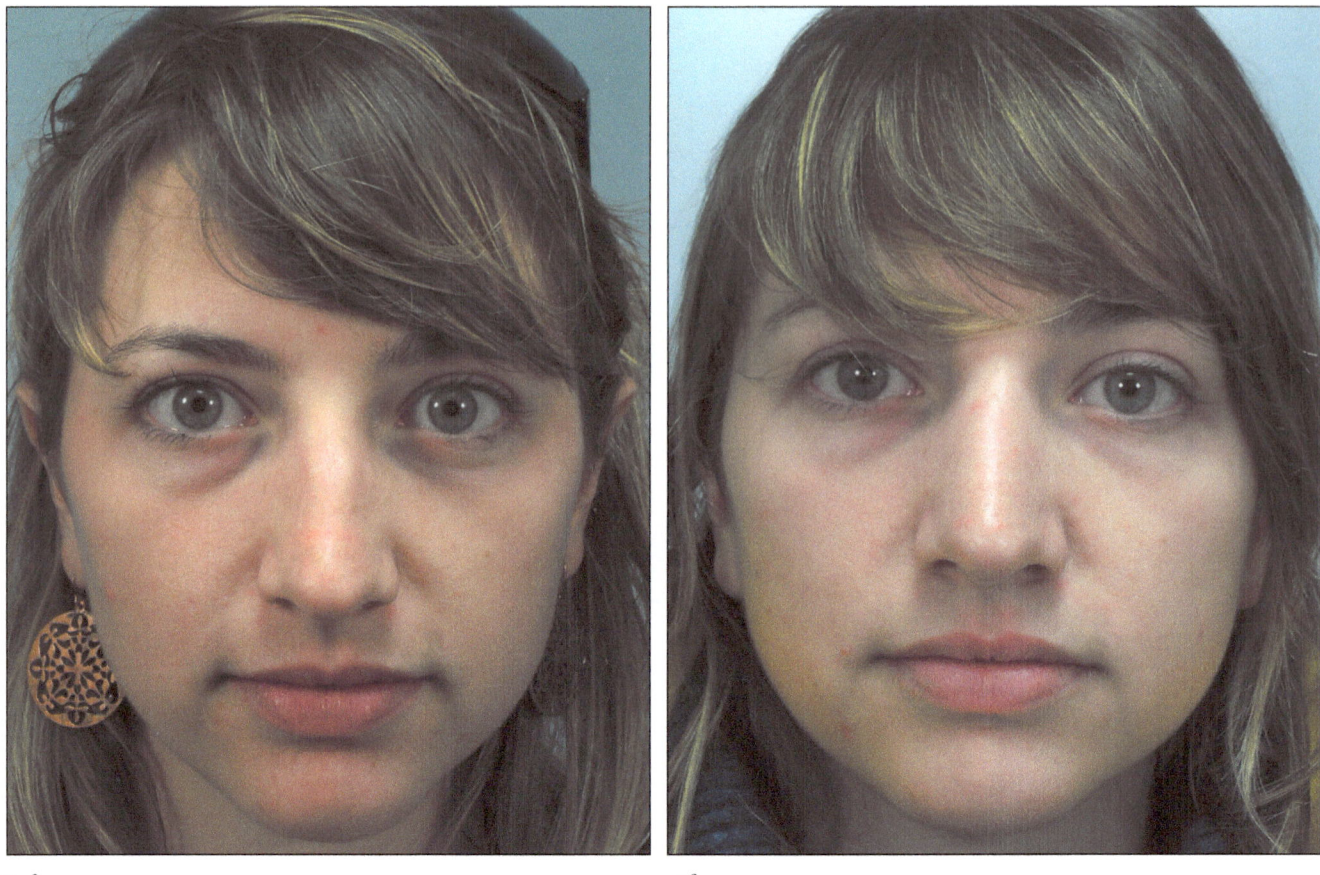

Before   *After*

NARROW MIDDLE VAULT, DORSAL BUMP, WITH SLIGHT OVERPROJECTION AND SLIGHT DROOPY TIP

This patient has a bump that is visible (as seen here and on the following on pages) and a narrow middle vault (middle section of nose). She also suffered from a chronic sinus disease and breathing difficulties and sought a subtle, natural improvement with rhinoplasty.

Rhinoplasty corrected her narrow middle vault and achieved a consistent width from top to bottom.

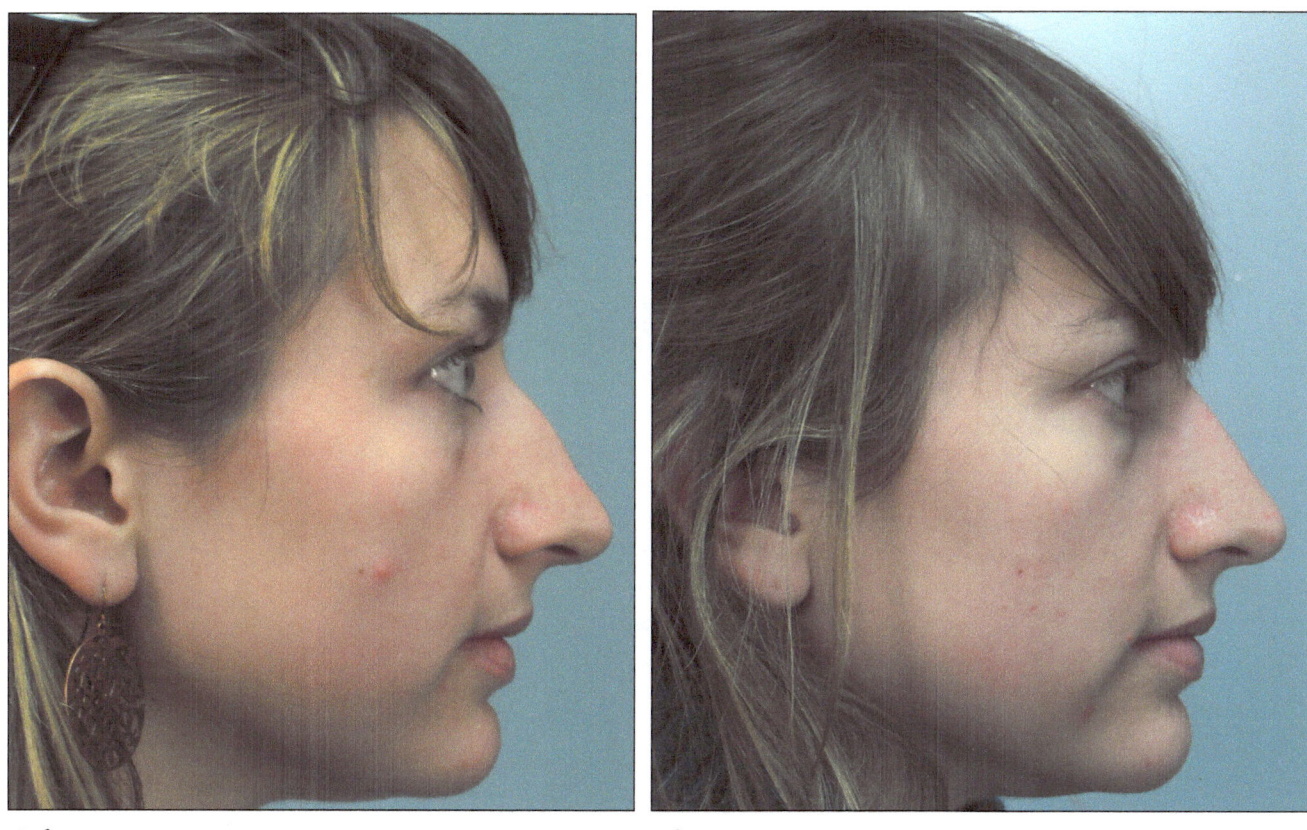

Before   *After*

NARROW MIDDLE VAULT, DORSAL BUMP, WITH SLIGHT OVERPROJECTION AND SLIGHT DROOPY TIP

It also reduced the projection of her nose and rotation of its tip upward slightly as seen here and on the following pages.

Now her nose is more in balance with other aspects of her face, resulting in a less harsh profile.

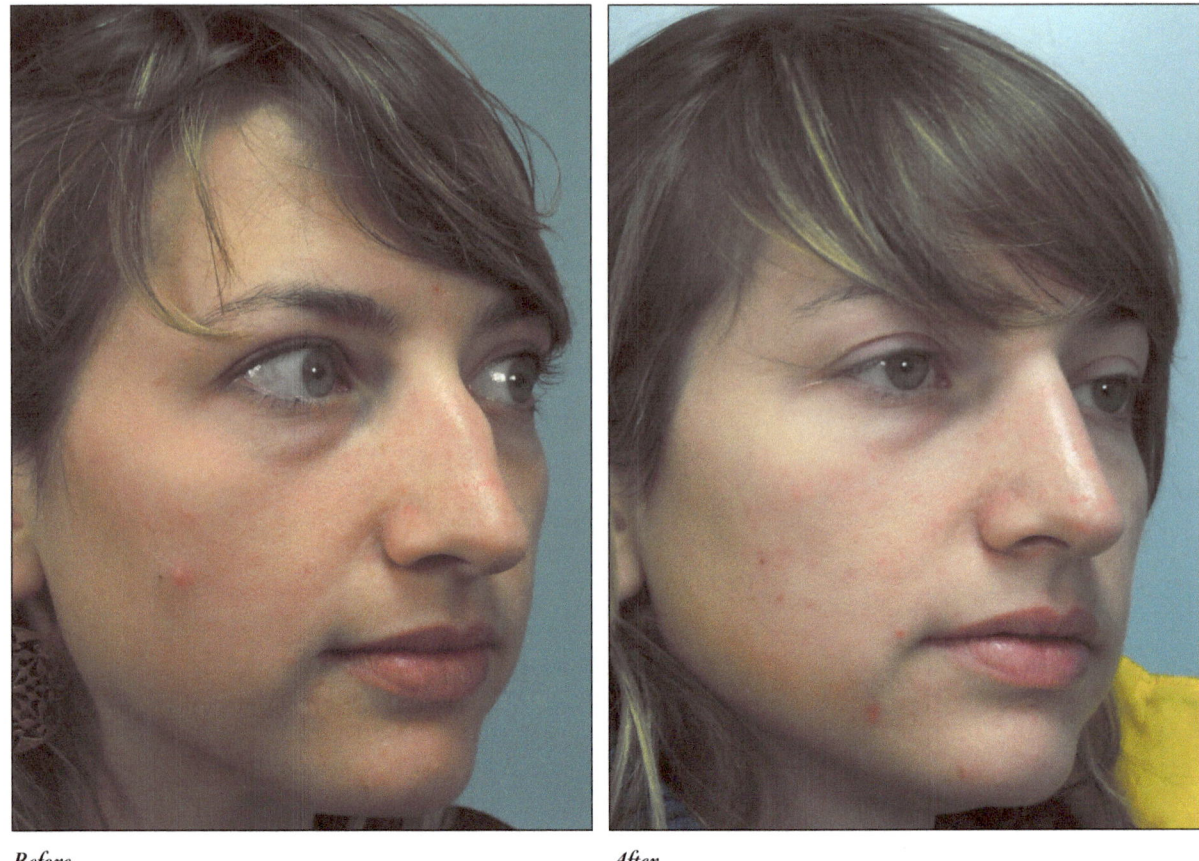

Before　　　　　　　　　　　　　　　　*After*

NARROW MIDDLE VAULT, DORSAL BUMP, WITH SLIGHT OVERPROJECTION AND SLIGHT DROOPY TIP

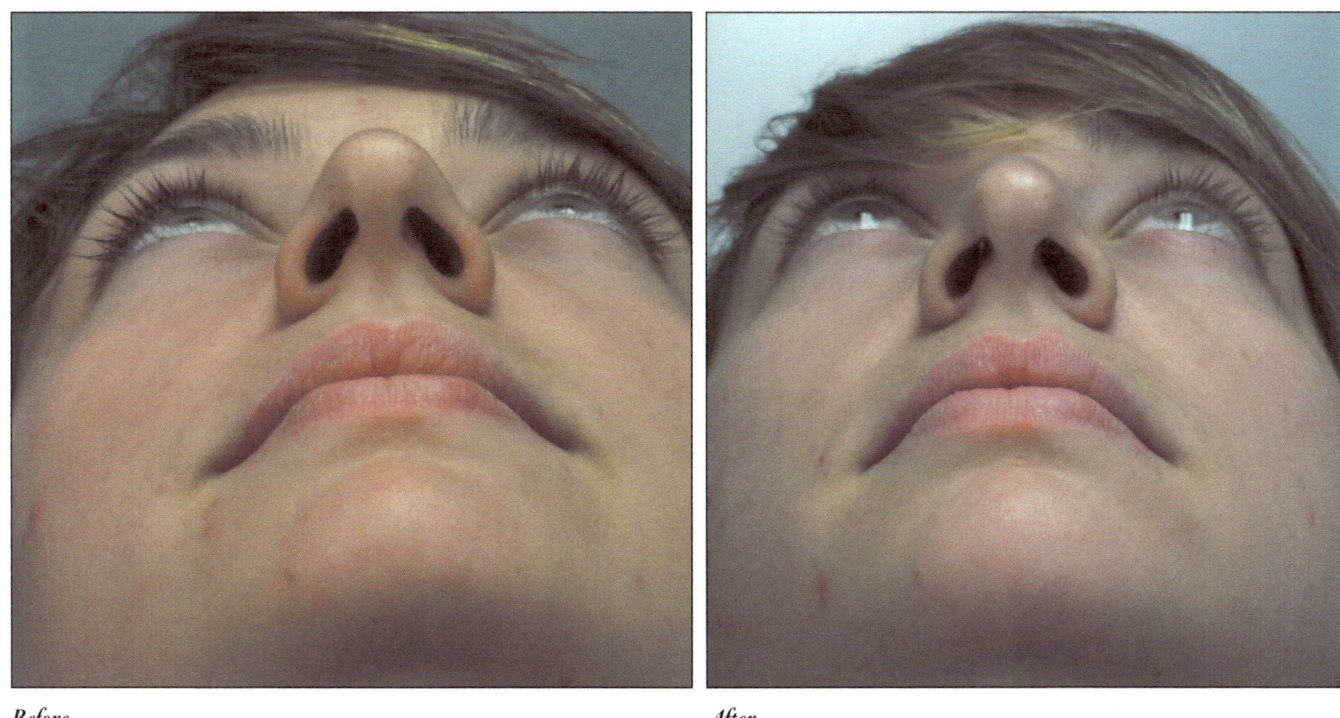

Before

After

NARROW MIDDLE VAULT, DORSAL BUMP, WITH SLIGHT OVERPROJECTION AND SLIGHT DROOPY TIP

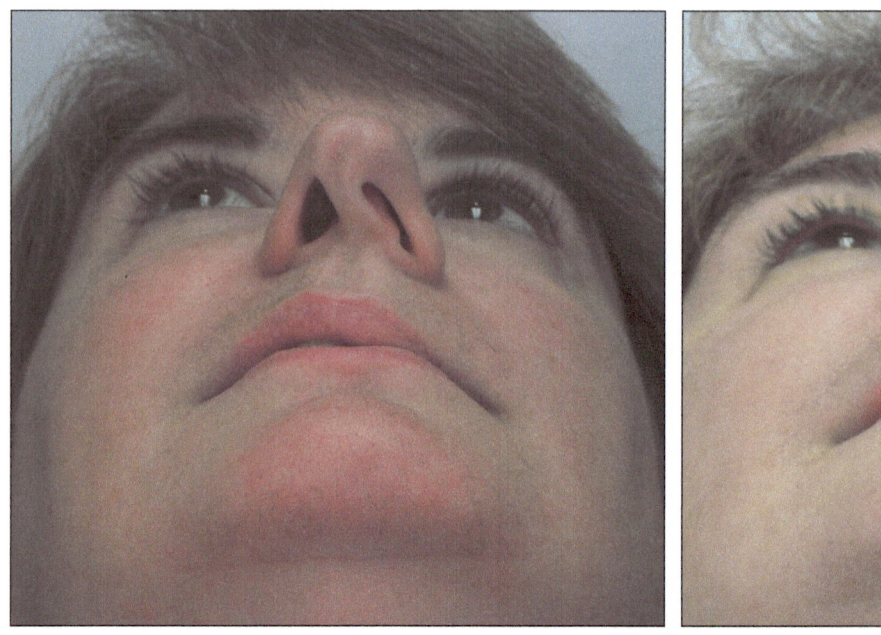
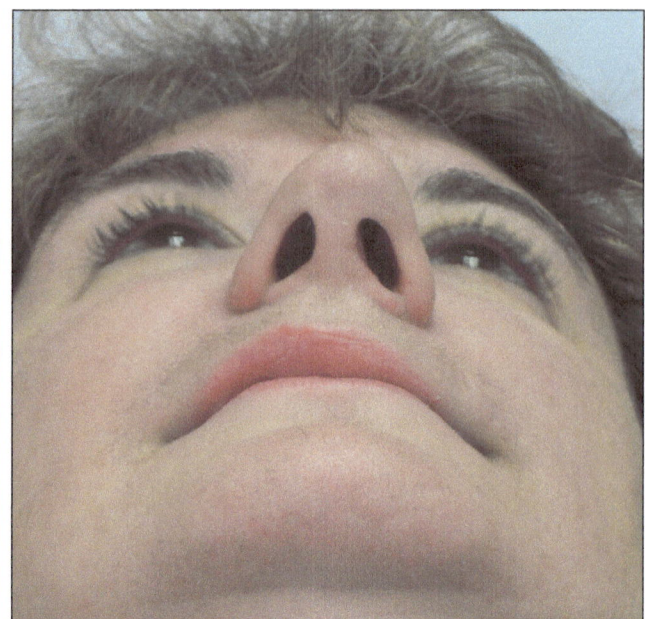

Before   *After*

CROOKED, TWISTED NOSE

This is a fairly common feature in a patient who is unable to breathe through her nose. She has a crooked, twisted nose. Rhinoplasty rebuilt the base of this patient's nose, correcting her breathing difficulty while giving her a more aesthetically pleasing nose.

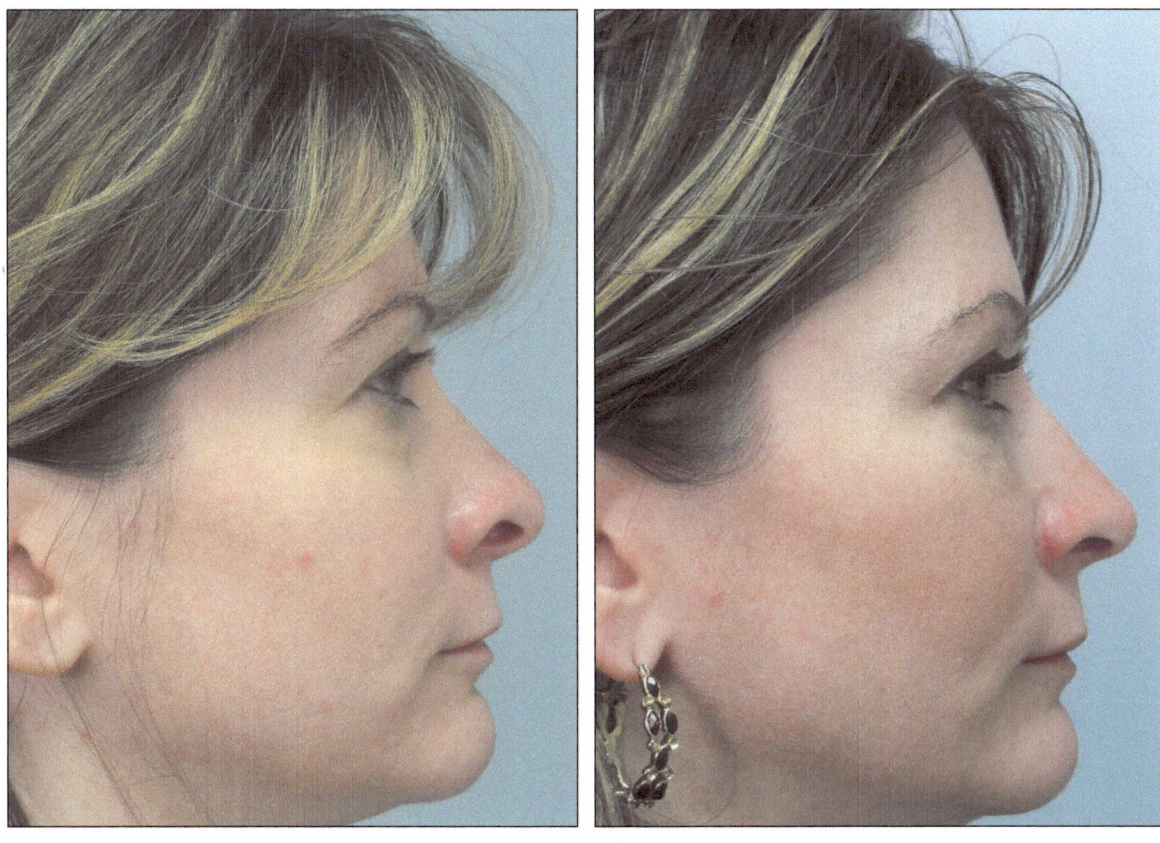

Before   *After*

NOTCHED NOSTRILS

This patient required a revision rhinoplasty that was due to having an excessive amount of cartilage removed from the nostril area. This drew attention to her nose by having anatomic features out of balance of what the eye expects.

Rhinoplasty involved a slight building up of the bridge of the nose and correcting the nostril notching.

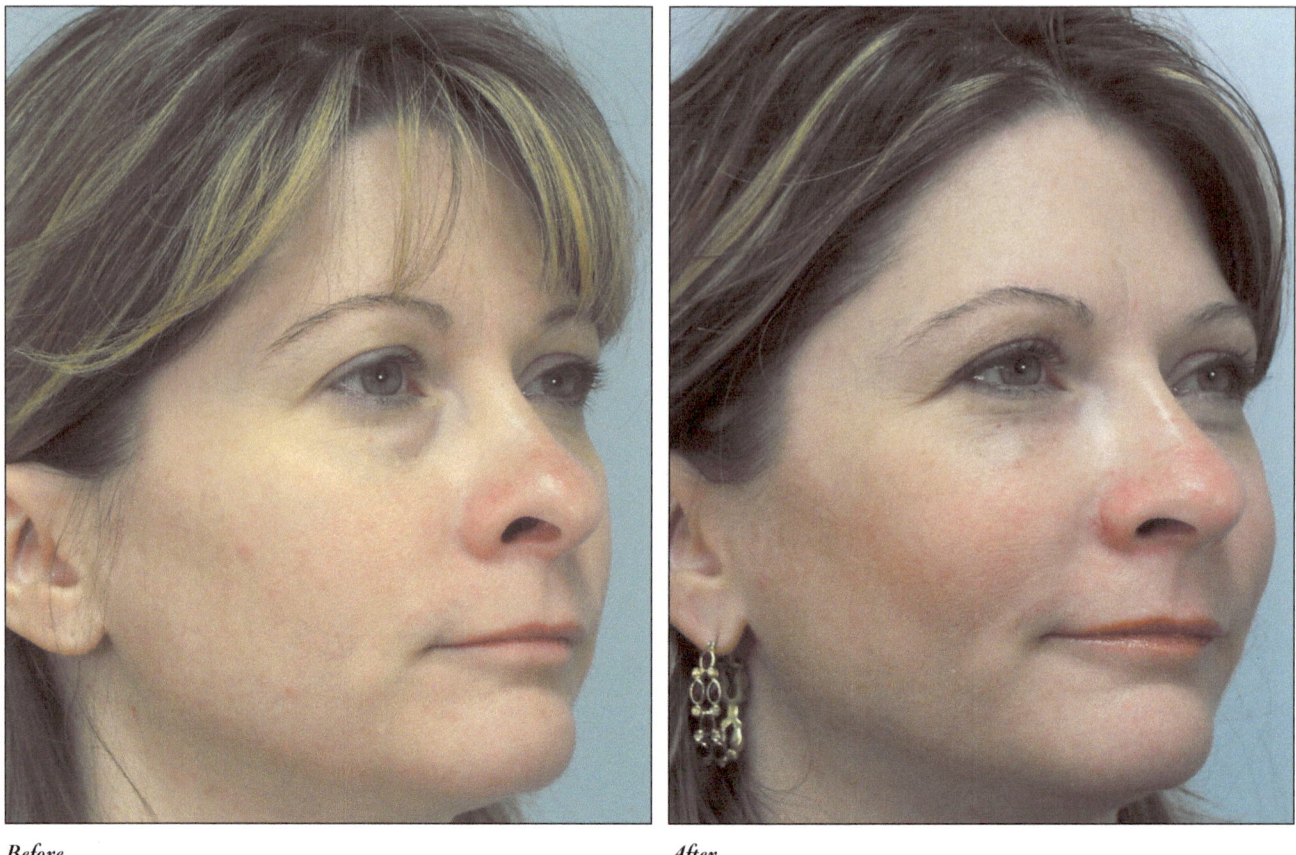

Before   *After*

NOTCHED NOSTRILS

The result of this subtle change is a more aesthetically pleasing nose that better fits the patient's face.

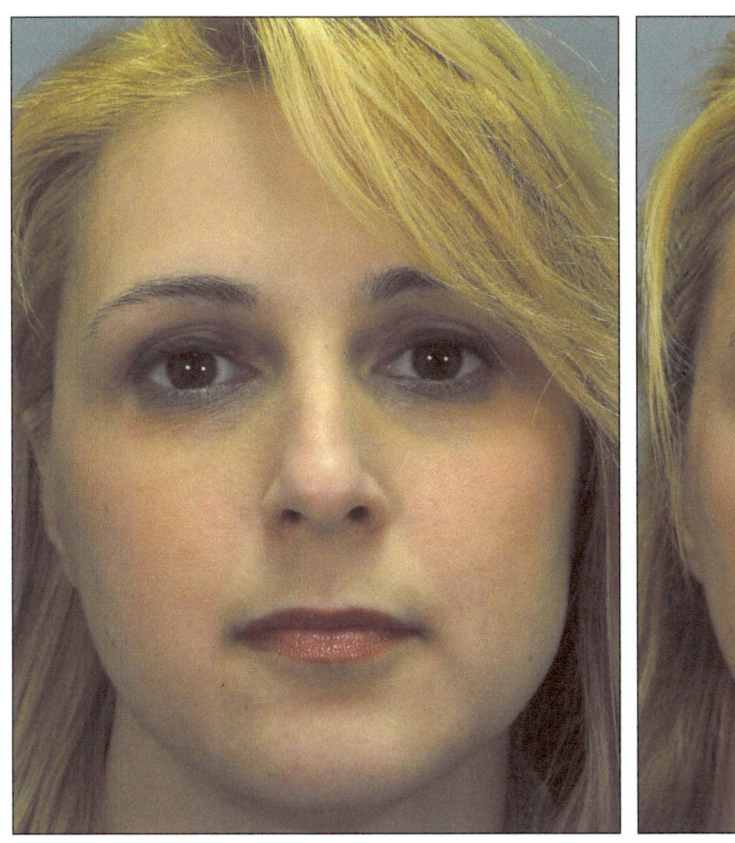

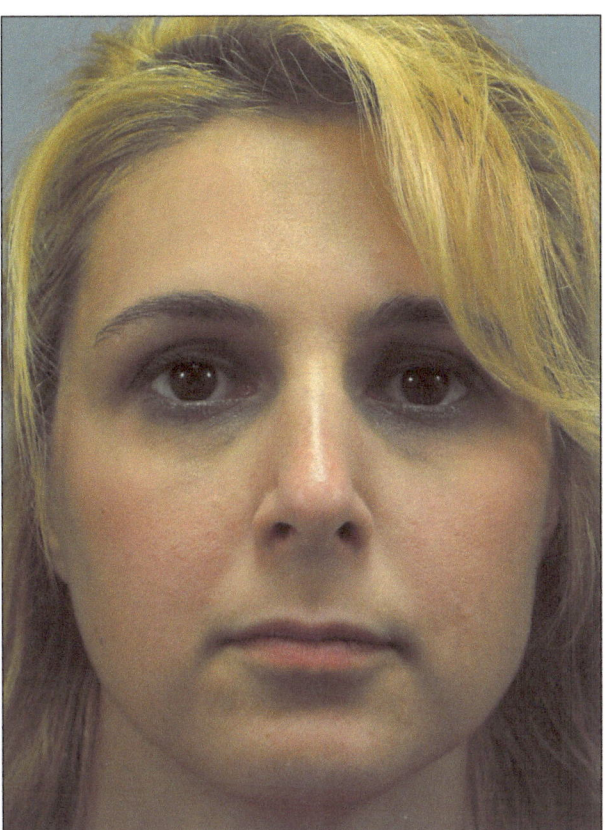

Before

After

LARGE BUMP WITH NARROW MIDDLE VAULT

The bump on this patient's nose has been reduced, which draws attention away from her profile toward her eyes. From the front view, the change is subtle, as the nose maintains its width from top to bottom and the tip is more refined. The result is a more pleasingly balanced face as seen on the following pages.

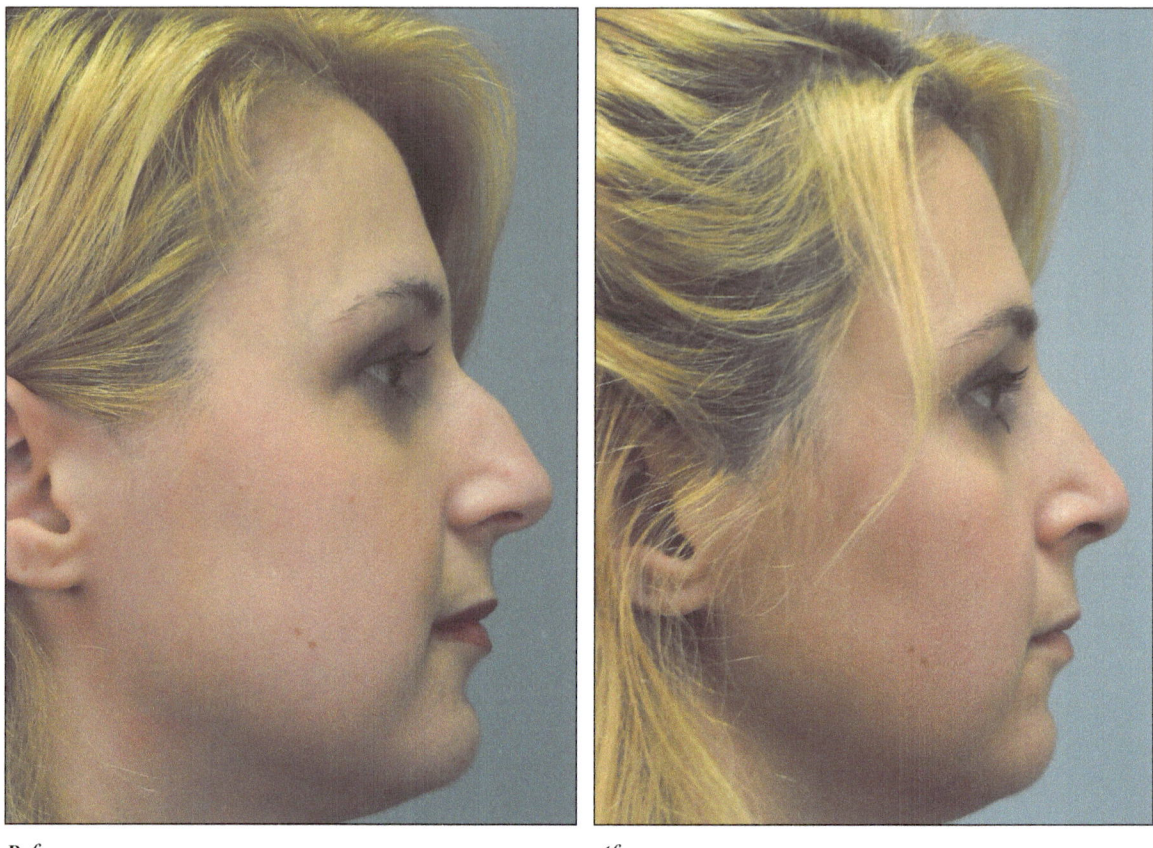

Before   *After*

LARGE BUMP WITH NARROW MIDDLE VAULT

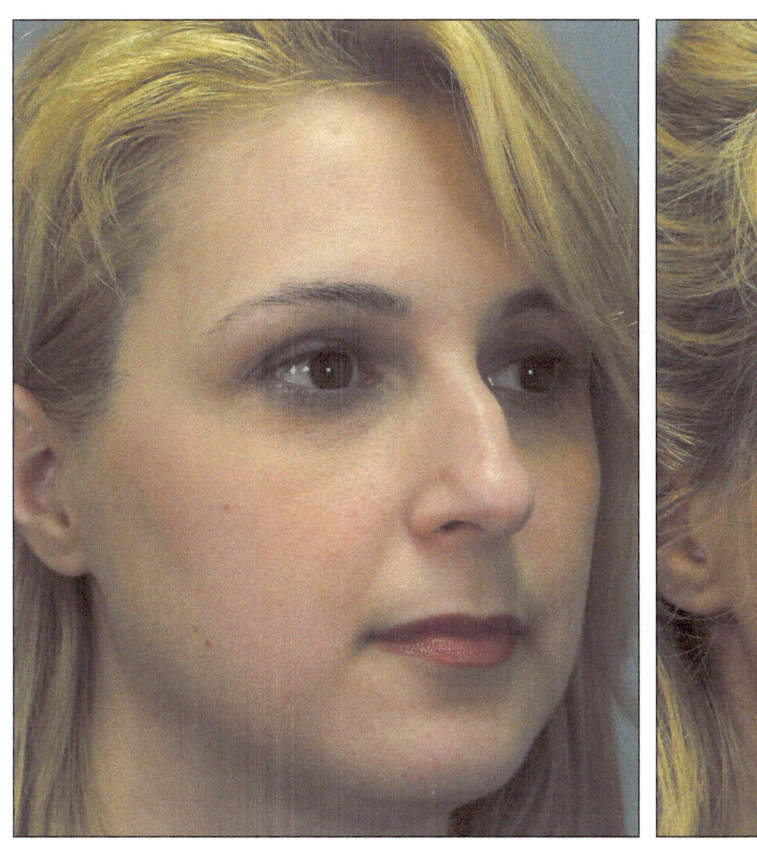

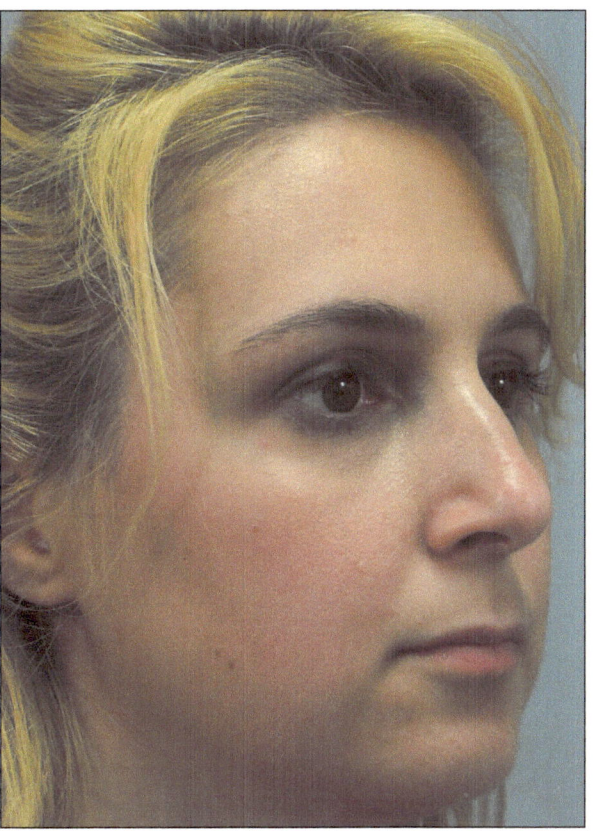

Before

After

LARGE BUMP WITH NARROW MIDDLE VAULT

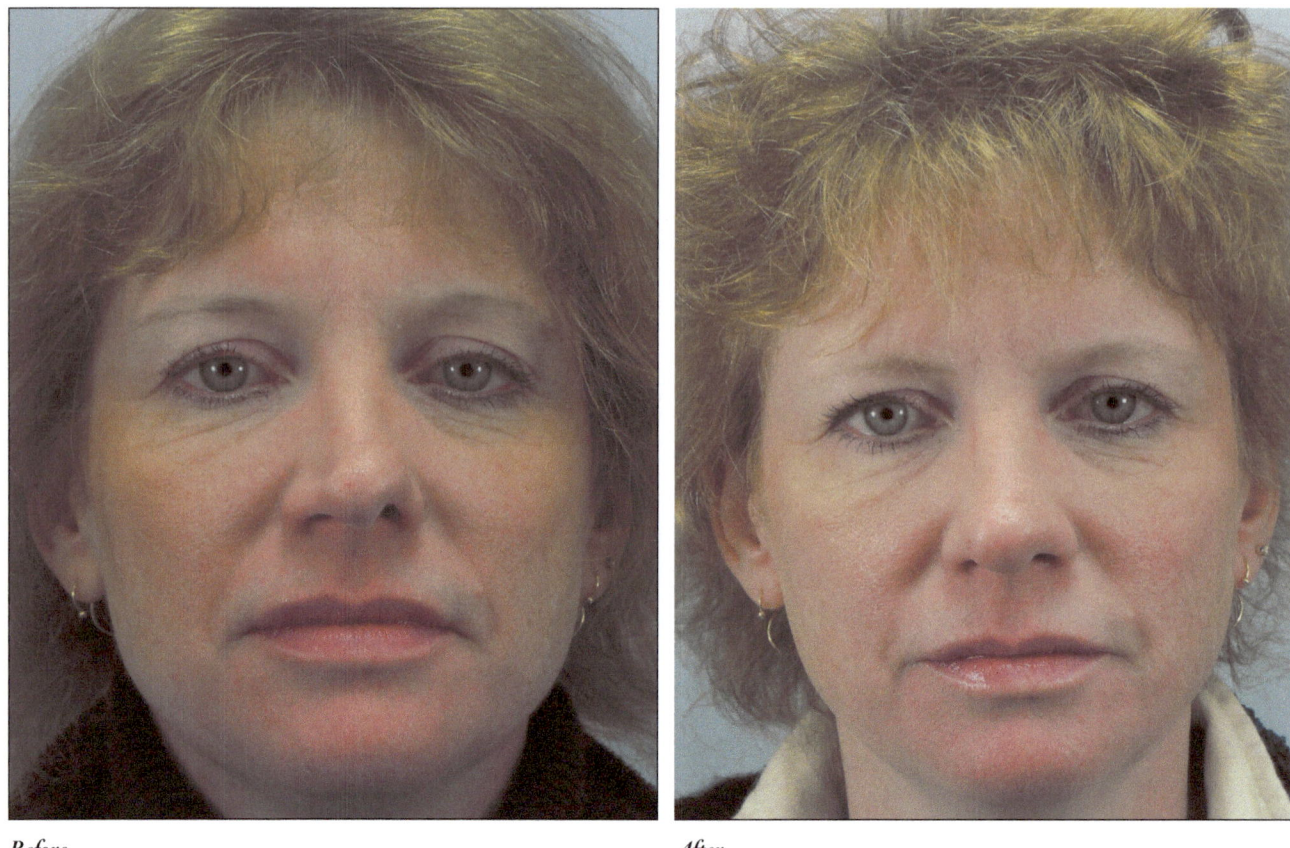

Before   *After*

PINCHED TIP AND CROOKED NASAL TIP WITH DIFFICULT BREATHING

This patient had difficulty breathing due to nasal wall collapse that disrupted her sleep and prevented her from feeling truly rested.

After rhinoplasty, her nose is straighter with more supported and symmetrical airways on both nostrils as seen above and on the following pages.

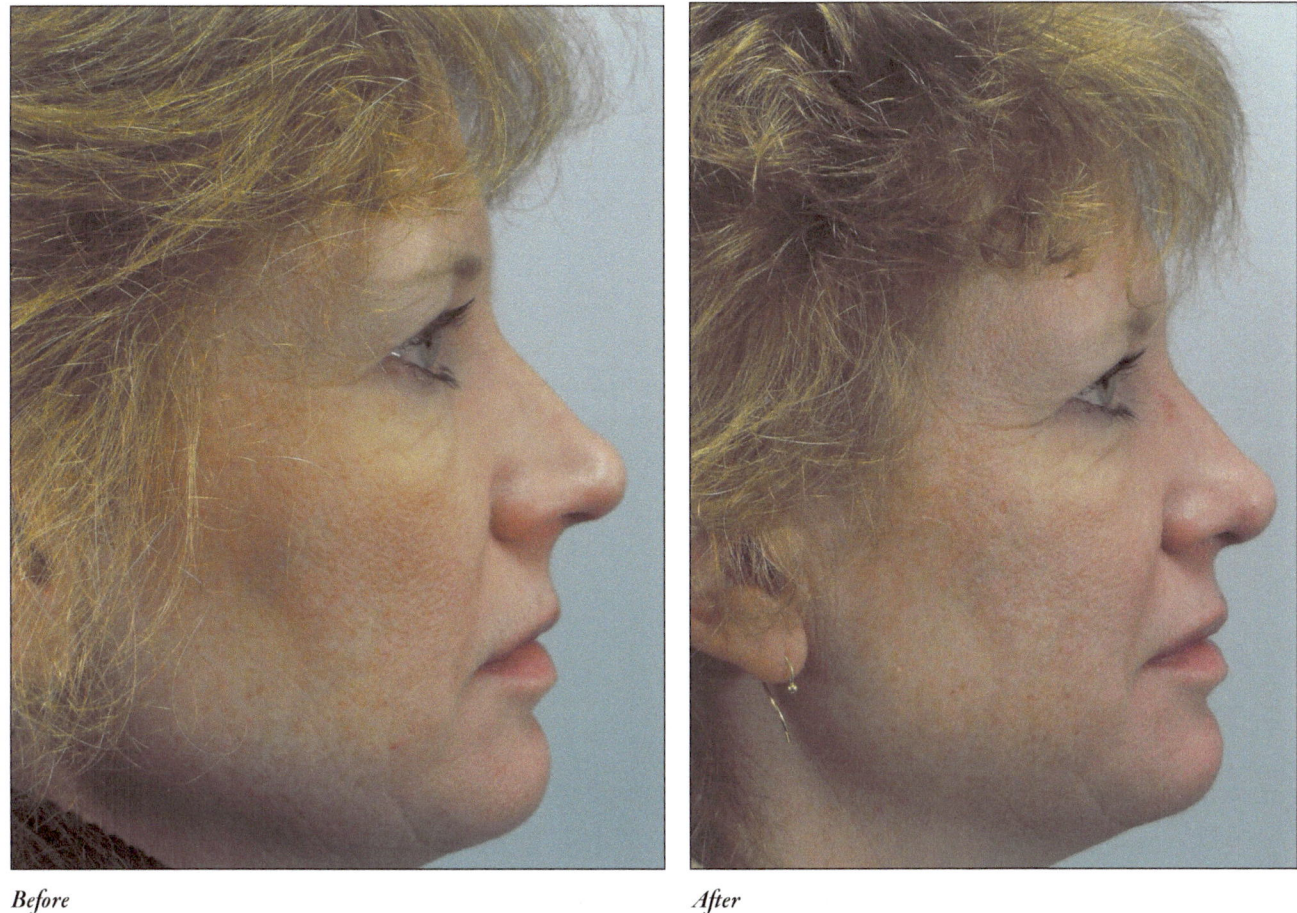

Before

After

PINCHED TIP AND CROOKED NASAL TIP WITH DIFFICULT BREATHING

Her collapsed nasal valve is now fixed, and she no longer experiences difficulty breathing. By reducing the size of her nasal tip and bringing this feature more in alignment with her face, we have also improved her profile.

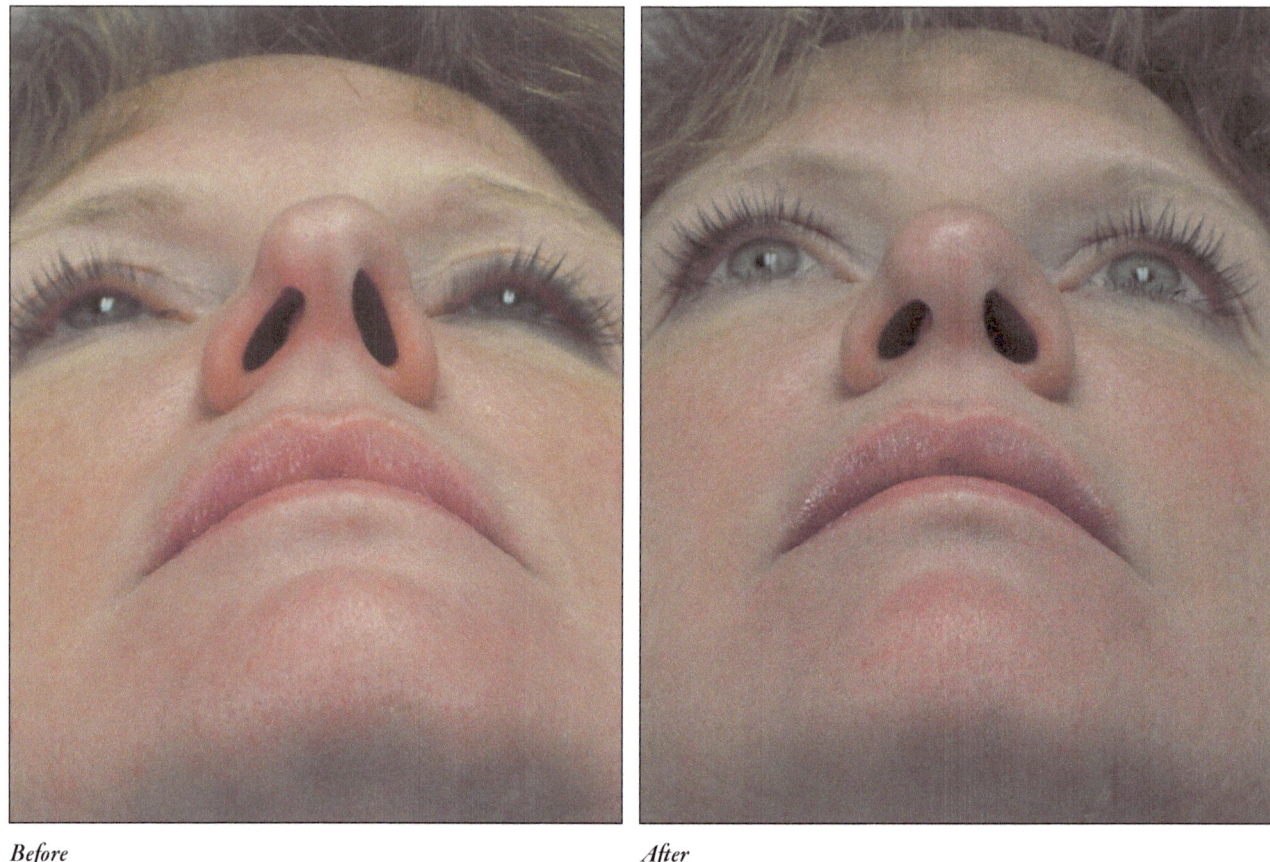

Before   *After*

PINCHED TIP AND CROOKED NASAL TIP WITH DIFFICULT BREATHING

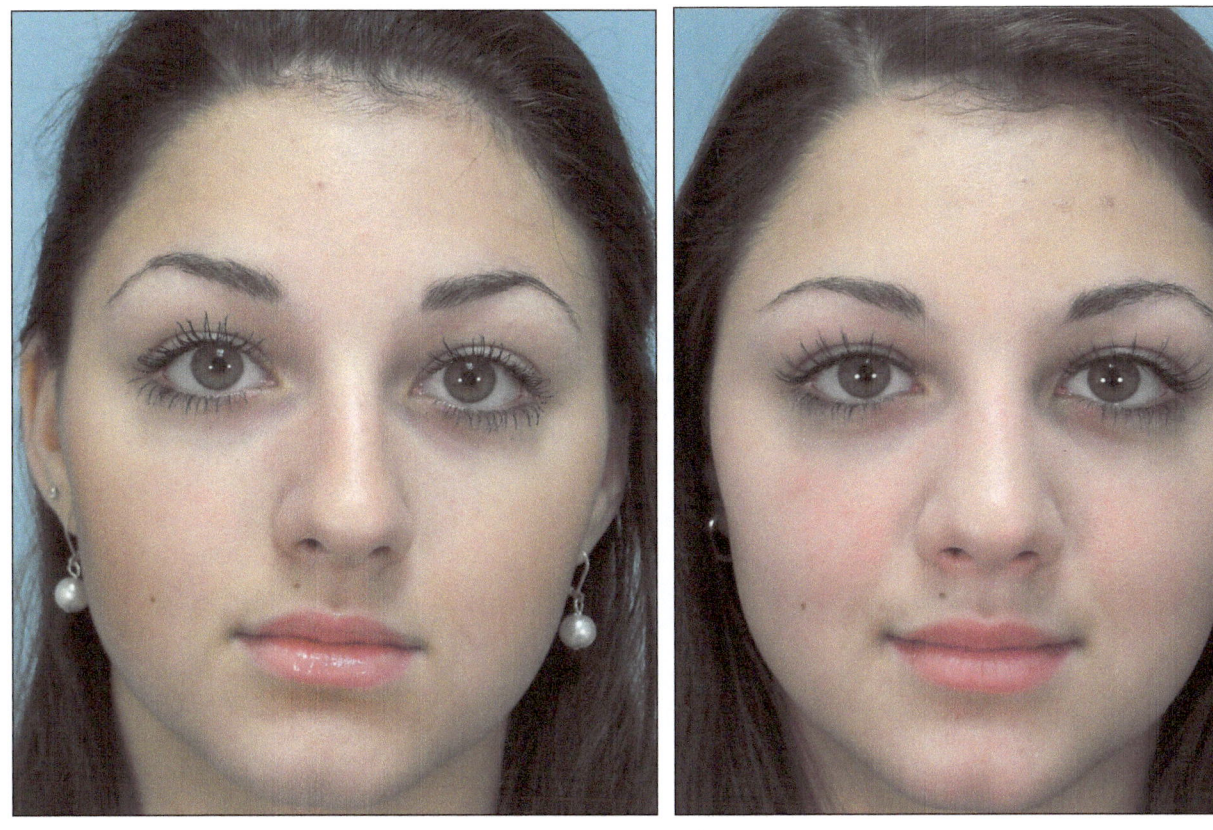

Before   *After*

SLIGHT DORSAL BUMP WITH DEVIATED SEPTUM

This patient had a problem breathing due to a deviated nasal septum. Also, she has a slight bump or dorsal convexity on her nose, giving her a more masculine look against her delicate features as seen above and on the following page.

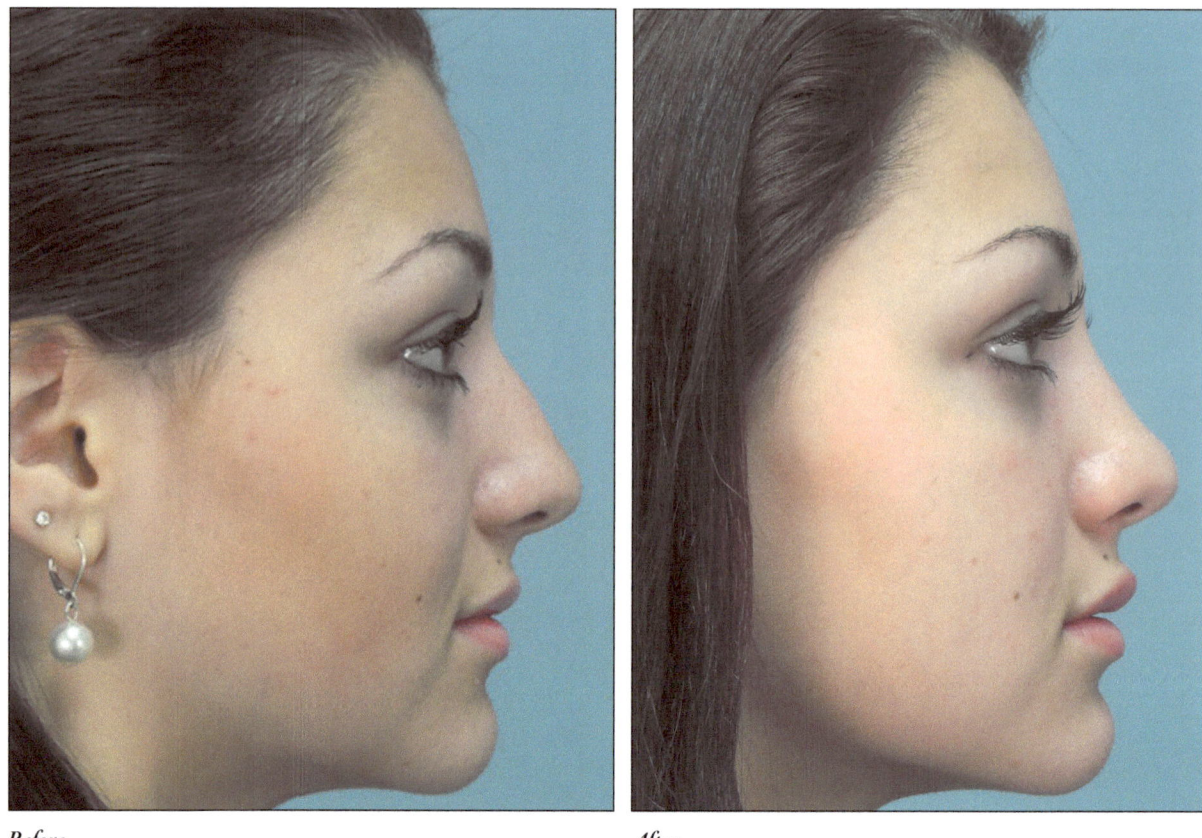

Before   *After*

SLIGHT DORSAL BUMP WITH DEVIATED SEPTUM

Rhinoplasty corrected her deviated septum and straightened and realigned her nose. Her nose is now aesthetically more pleasing, feminine, and befitting her face as seen here and on the following pages.

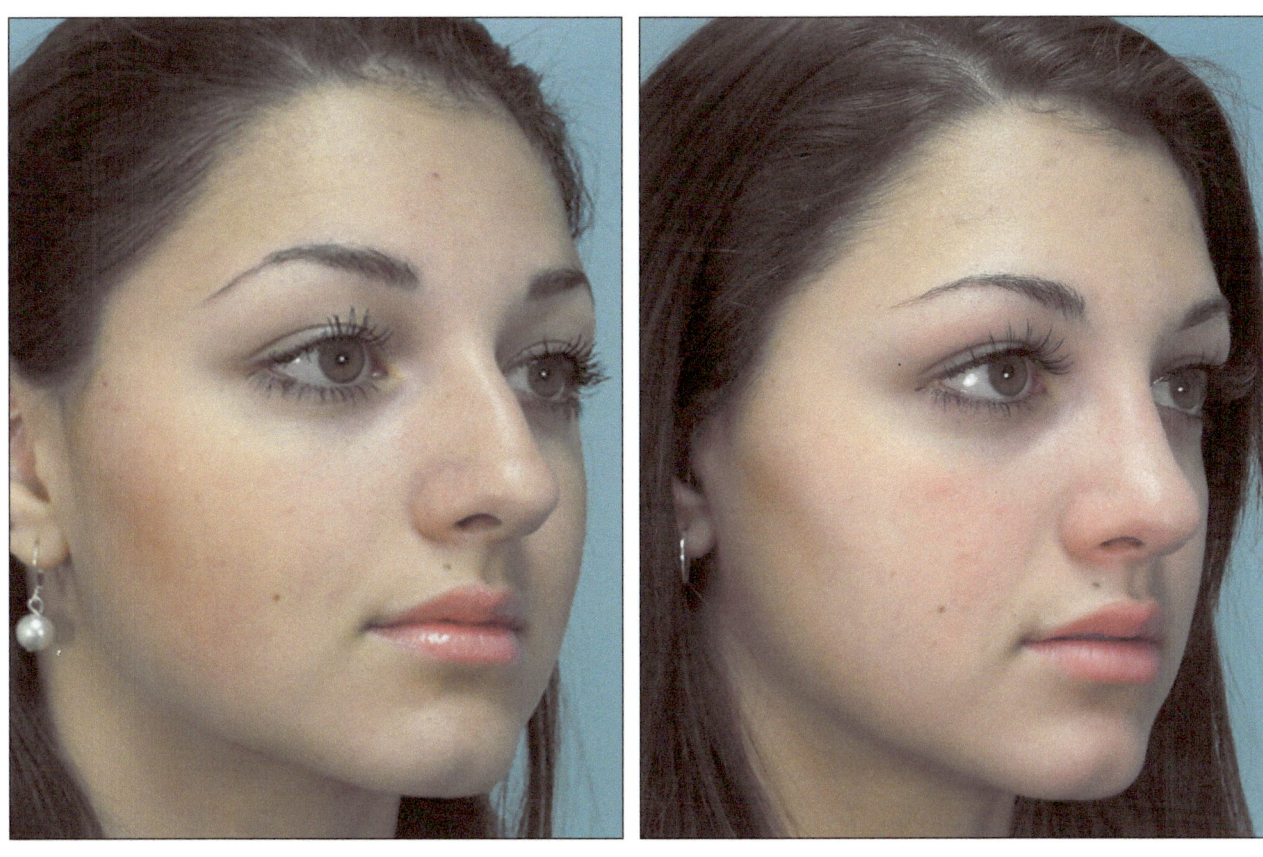

Before

After

SLIGHT DORSAL BUMP WITH DEVIATED SEPTUM

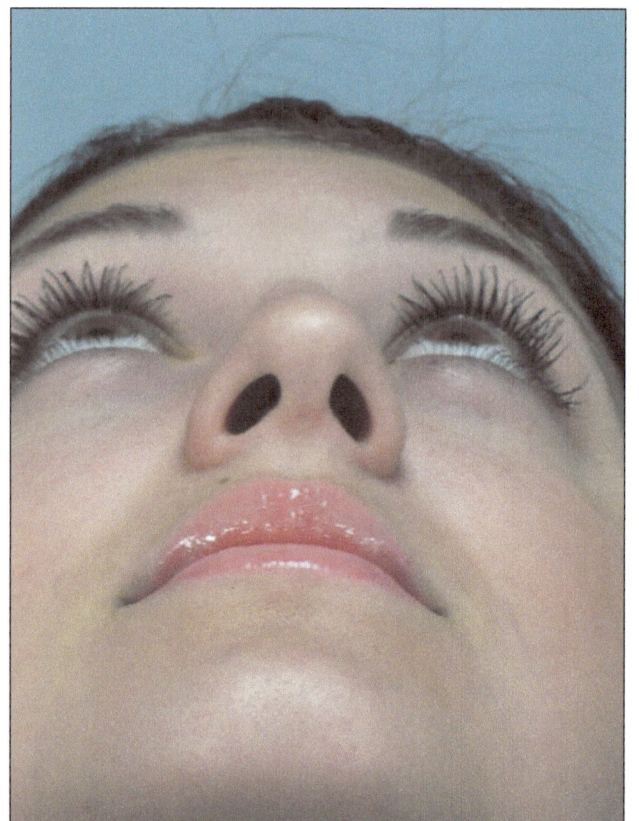

Before

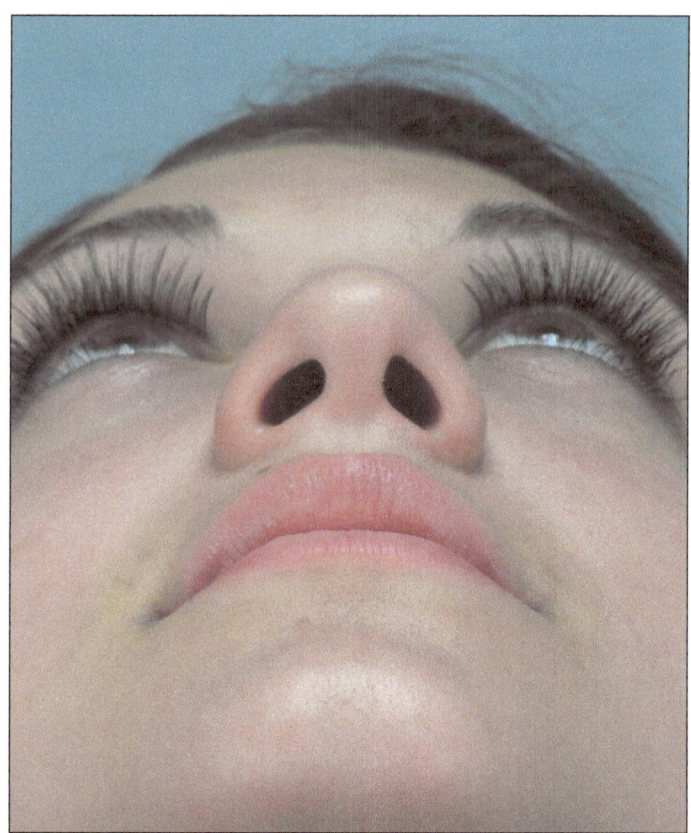

After

SLIGHT DORSAL BUMP WITH DEVIATED SEPTUM

http://www.youtube.com/watch?v=NM2N9hSB8R0&list=PL4CDA45694188ABB0&index=60